Concept Development in Nursing

Foundations, Techniques, and Applications

BETH L. RODGERS, RN, PhD

Associate Professor, School of Nursing
University of Wisconsin—Milwaukee
Milwaukee, Wisconsin

KATHLEEN A. KNAFL, PhD

Professor, College of Nursing
University of Illinois at Chicago
Chicago, Illinois

W.B. SAUNDERS COMPANY
A Division of Harcourt Brace & Company
PHILADELPHIA   LONDON   TORONTO   MONTREAL   SYDNEY   TOKYO

W.B. SAUNDERS COMPANY
A Division of
Harcourt Brace & Company

The Curtis Center
Independence Square West
Philadelphia, Pennsylvania 19106

Library of Congress Cataloging-in-Publication Data
Concept development in nursing : foundations, techniques, and applications / [edited by] Beth L. Rodgers, Kathleen A. Knafl.

Concept development in nursing : foundations, techniques, and
  applications / [edited by] Beth L. Rodgers, Kathleen A. Knafl.
      p.   cm.
    Includes bibliographical references.
    ISBN 0–7216–3674–8
      1. Nursing—Philosophy.   2. Concepts.   I. Rodgers, Beth L.
  II. Knafl, Kathleen Astin.
      [DNLM: 1. Concept Formation.   2. Nursing.   WY 86 C7435 1993]
  RT84.5.C6624   1993
  610.73'01—dc20
  DNLM/DLC   93–7421

CONCEPT DEVELOPMENT IN NURSING:
Foundations, Techniques, and Applications   ISBN 0-7216-3674-8

Printed in United States of America

Last digit is the print number   9 8 7 6 5 4 3 2 1

Contributors

CYNTHIA ALLEN ABBOTT, RN, PhD, CNOR
MAJ(P) Army Nurse Corps, University of Texas at Austin, Austin, Texas
Wilsonian Concept Analysis: Applying the Technique

KAY C. AVANT, RN, PhD, FAAN
Associate Professor, University of Texas at Austin, School of Nursing,
Austin, Texas
*The Wilson Method of Concept Analysis; Wilsonian Concept Analysis:
Applying the Technique*

TERESA BRITT, RN, MS
Case Management Supervisor, Carle Clinical Studies, Champaign, Illinois
*Simultaneous Concept Analysis: A Strategy for Developing Multiple
Interrelated Concepts*

MARION E. BROOME, RN, PhD
Professor, College of Nursing, Rush University; Assistant Chairperson,
Maternal-Child Department, Rush—Presbyterian—St. Luke's Medical
Center, Chicago, Illinois
Integrative Literature Reviews in the Development of Concepts

DOROTHY D. CAMILLERI, RN, PhD
Assistant Professor, College of Nursing, University of Illinois at Chicago,
Chicago, Illinois
Concept Development in Nursing Diagnosis

DORIS D. COWARD, RN, PhD
Assistant Professor, School of Nursing, University of Texas at Austin,
Austin, Texas
*Simultaneous Concept Analysis: A Strategy for Developing Multiple
Interrelated Concepts*

KATHLEEN V. COWLES, RN, PhD
Associate Professor, School of Nursing, University of Wisconsin—
Milwaukee, Milwaukee, Wisconsin
The Concept of Grief: An Evolutionary Perspective

NANCY S. CREASON, RN, PhD
Dean and Professor, School of Nursing, Southern Illinois University at
Edwardsville, Edwardsville, Illinois
Concept Development in Nursing Diagnosis

JANET A. DEATRICK, RN, PhD, FAAN
Associate Professor and Program Director, Nursing of Children Graduate
Program, School of Nursing, University of Pennsylvania, Philadelphia,
Pennsylvania
Knowledge Synthesis and Concept Development in Nursing

JOAN E. HAASE, RN, PhD
Assistant Professor, College of Nursing, University of Arizona, Tucson,
Arizona
*Simultaneous Concept Analysis: A Strategy for Developing Multiple
Interrelated Concepts*

HESOOK SUZIE KIM, RN, PhD
Professor, College of Nursing, University of Rhode Island, Kingston,
Rhode Island
*An Expansion and Elaboration of the Hybrid Model of Concept
Development*

MI JA KIM, RN, PhD, FAAN
Professor and Dean, College of Nursing, University of Illinois at Chicago,
Chicago, Illinois
Concept Development in Nursing Diagnosis

KATHLEEN A. KNAFL, PhD
Professor, College of Nursing, University of Illinois at Chicago, Chicago,
Illinois
*Introduction to Concept Development in Nursing; Knowledge Synthesis
and Concept Development in Nursing; Applications and Future
Directions for Concept Development in Nursing*

NANCY R. LACKEY, RN, PhD
Associate Professor, College of Nursing, University of Tennessee,
Memphis, Tennessee
Concept Clarification: Using the Norris Method in Clinical Research

NANCY KLINE LEIDY, RN, PhD
Senior Staff Fellow, National Center for Nursing Research, Division of
Intramural Research, Laboratory for the Study of Human Responses to
Health and Illness, National Institutes of Health, Bethesda, Maryland
*Simultaneous Concept Analysis: A Strategy for Developing Multiple
Interrelated Concepts*

PATRICIA E. PENN, PhD
Senior Research Specialist, Department of Psychology, University of
Arizona; Clinical Research Psychologist, La Frontera Center, Tucson,
Arizona
*Simultaneous Concept Analysis: A Strategy for Developing Multiple
Interrelated Concepts*

BETH L. RODGERS, RN, PhD
Associate Professor, School of Nursing, University of Wisconsin—
Milwaukee, Milwaukee, Wisconsin
*Introduction to Concept Development in Nursing; Philosophical
Foundations of Concept Development; Concept Analysis: An
Evolutionary View; The Concept of Grief: An Evolutionary Perspective;
Applications and Future Directions for Concept Development in
Nursing*

DONNA SCHWARTZ-BARCOTT, RN, PhD
Professor and Director of Graduate Studies, College of Nursing, University
of Rhode Island, Kingston, Rhode Island
*An Expansion and Elaboration of the Hybrid Model of Concept
Development; A Concept Analysis of Withdrawal: Application of the
Hybrid Model of Concept Development*

GERALDINE VERHULST, RN, MSN
Assistant Professor of Nursing, Rhode Island College, Providence, Rhode
Island
*A Concept Analysis of Withdrawal: Application of the Hybrid Model of
Concept Development*

Preface

$\mathcal{B}$eginnings and endings (like concepts) can be elusive to pinpoint. Although we can identify the time when we first discussed the possibility of collaborating on a book on concept development, the origins of our individual and shared interests in concept analysis and concept development in general are considerably less clear. The idea for the book was first broached at the 1990 conference of the Midwest Nursing Research Society (MNRS). We each had been a presenter at a symposium on concept analysis, and following the symposium a mutual friend suggested that we collaborate on a book on the subject. Rodgers had mulled over the idea of such a project for some time, and the prospect of working with Knafl, of sharing ideas and enthusiasm, as well as expertise, was an added impetus. The idea of working together appealed to both of us, and over the course of several conversations and planning sessions we developed an outline and prospectus to show to possible publishers. Although that first meeting at MNRS was the official beginning of the project, our individual interests in concept development go back much further.

Rodgers has a history of fondness for analytical pursuits, scholarly questioning, and the abstract. In the 1980s, however, prompted by graduate study, this attraction focused on the nature of nursing and the many issues and problems encountered in attempts to develop the knowledge base of nursing. Philosophical pursuits quickly made it clear that many of the problems confronted in nursing were conceptual. This observation led to further inquiry to seek credible means to resolve these barriers.

Concept analysis had been used with some frequency to address such problems in nursing. Yet in the nursing literature this method was limited to a few approaches that were similar in orientation. Existing descriptions provided little insight into elements of rigor associated with analysis, how methodological decisions were made, or specifically how using a particular method could advance nursing knowledge. On close examination there also was reason for concern regarding potential conflict between the philosophical basis implicit in the literature and the contemporary philosophy and beliefs espoused in nursing. Ultimately this led Rodgers to investigate various nursing and philosophical positions on concepts in general, to consider a variety of means to resolve conceptual problems, and to explore the linkage between concepts and nursing knowledge.

In contrast to the philosophical groundings of Rodgers' interests, as a family researcher Knafl was interested in the potential inherent in concepts for increasing understanding of family response to illness. She also was aware of the conceptual ambiguity surrounding many of the concepts used in family research (e.g., family coping, enmeshment) but accepted this as a "fact of life." This acceptance changed rather abruptly after she read the concept analysis section of the first edition of Chinn and Jacobs' book on theory development in nursing. For Knafl the book raised an intellectual challenge and presented a strategy for addressing some of the intellectual ambiguity in family research.

For several years, Knafl and her colleague Janet Deatrick had puzzled over the meaning of two concepts, normalization and denial, that often were used to describe parents' responses to their child's chronic illness. During the course of their work with families of children with chronic illness, Knafl and Deatrick had noted that occasionally families they described as normalizing their children's illnesses were described by providers as denying the seriousness of the situations. Knafl and Deatrick knew that they wanted to do something to clarifiy this conceptual confusion, but it was not until they read about concept analysis that they found an appropriate strategy to pursue. In 1984 they published their first concept analysis of normalization. A second analysis of the concept of family management style was published several years later. In the course of completing these analyses and reading more on concept analysis, Knafl and Deatrick became aware of other approaches to concept analysis and development that raised numerous questions about the relative merits and appropriate use of these alternative strategies. Rodgers' philosophical interest in these field provided the ideal complement to Knafl's more applied interest in concept development.

This book reflects our complementary interests. In it, we address both the philosophical underpinnings of concept development and the practicality of various techniques for furthering understanding and progress in important areas of nursing science. Further, we have included an encompassing range of concept development strategies and discussed the advantages, disadvantages, and, most importantly, the appropriate use of each. We see the book as providing a menu of possibilities for all those in nursing who are interested in contributing to the further clarification and development of the many concepts pertinent to nursing practice, research, and education.

Many people have influenced this work, both directly and indirectly, and we would like to acknowledge their roles in the creation of this text. First, we must acknowledge the contributions of previous authors who have written on the subject of concepts and concept development. In a field such as nursing where inquiry easily becomes focused primarily on the empirical realm, we are grateful for those thinkers and authors in the past who pointed out the importance of conceptual concerns in the advancement of nursing. Their works not only have contributed to our own thinking about this subject matter but also undoubtedly have helped to set the stage for this text, which we expect to represent the current state of the science of concept development.

We also want to acknowledge the contributing authors, who enthusiastically shared their expertise for this project and thus provided the support essential to make our plans and ideas for this book a reality. Kathleen Cowles provided much of the initial impetus for this work through her unfaltering belief that it was, indeed, a worthwhile pursuit and by being the catalyst in encouraging our collaboration on this project. Janet Deatrick contributed her valuable insights and spirit of adventure to Knafl's initial forays into the realm of concept analysis. Finally, we wish to acknowledge and express our gratitude to the staff of W. B. Saunders Company, all of whom were nothing short of terrific to work with. Mr. Thomas Eoyang, Editor-in-Chief, deserves special recognition for "sticking his neck out" to support what some might consider a rather esoteric work. We also would like to acknowledge Mary Espenchied of CRACOM who provided exceptional editing work, along with the many others responsible for turning our ideas into this printed volume.

We want to point out here that any reference to this book as a "finished" product must be considered again in regard to the elusiveness of beginnings and endings, as we noted at the opening of this preface. There is good reason to argue whether scholarly work and inquiry are ever truly "finished." Instead, it seems that we reach transition stages where it is worthwhile and important to share ideas and information garnered but equally important to stimulate further inquiry. Consequently, we consider this book not as an end product, but as a beginning. We hope that it can serve as the catalyst to stimulate further dialogue and work on concept development in nursing.

BETH L. RODGERS
KATHLEEN A. KNAFL

Contents

Chapter 1

Introduction to Concept Development in Nursing

BETH L. RODGERS AND KATHLEEN A. KNAFL

*S*ome readers of this book, at first glance, may have the same type of reaction that many of our colleagues did when they first heard of our project: "Hmmm. Sounds interesting." This is a classic, noncommittal response that, since it frequently is accompanied by a puzzled expression, conveys that the speaker really does not know what to think. Most likely, they really were wondering "What is concept development, anyway, and what does it have to do with nursing (and why should anyone care)?" We had heard these questions many times before. Certainly, there were many people who responded to our idea for this text with excitement and anticipation. This wide variety of reactions, which we both had encountered through our experiences with research, publishing, and giving presentations, provided much of the motivation for this work. We hope that it will answer at least some of the questions of the curious or puzzled, provide stimulation for those already excited about prospects for concept development for the advancement of nursing knowledge, and promote greater understanding of the depth and scope of concept development in nursing for all readers.

For the uninitiated, we aimed to provide information that would answer the "what is it?" (and, hopefully, the "who cares?") question. We also wanted to stimulate interest in concept development methods as a part of the readers' own research programs or, at least, an appreciation of such inquiry. For the reader who has had some exposure to ideas related to concept development but lacks sufficient background to tackle this type of investigation, we have assembled a combination of how-to descriptions, along with practical examples and additional discussion on applications. The intent here also was to provide sufficient background information and rationale to promote investigations that would be both rigorous and credible. Too often, concept development techniques seem to be relegated to the status of classroom learning exercises; thus, their place and contributions in the realm of nursing knowledge development may not be appreciated fully. Finally, for the advanced reader, we tried to create a text that is comprehensive, presenting views and discussions that either were not available elsewhere, were available only in less depth or lesser states of development, or were more or less obscure by virtue of being scattered throughout existing literature. By assembling a wide variety of concept development approaches and applications in a single text, the differences across methods become more apparent. An understanding of diverse approaches is necessary for the researcher to make informed choices in selecting a technique to employ in an investigation.

Concept development is not a new area or system of methods for inquiry. Books and articles on research methods and theory building are abundant, and occasionally include some attention to ideas related to concept development. Typically this attention is focused on concepts in general, particularly in texts related to theory or, in some cases, a discussion of concept analysis as a method. These efforts do not capture the scope or depth of the topic of concept development, nor do they adequately emphasize the contribution of concept development in the overall scientific enterprise of nursing.

The lack of concentrated attention to this topic is particularly troublesome in view of the overall importance of concepts in the development of knowledge. In the literature on research methods, the conceptual basis for a study often is discussed as the hallmark (or, in some cases, the primary failing point) of excellence in an investigation. In theory development literature, concepts are widely recognized as the "building blocks" from which theories are constructed. In philosophy, there is a lengthy history of discussions of science and knowledge. Without variation, concepts are a major focus for the majority, if not all, of these writers.

This emphasis on concepts has increased somewhat in recent years. Predominant philosophers of science in the early twentieth century, particularly the logical positivists, confined conceptual problems to the realm of "nonsense." More recently, however, philosophers such as Laudan (1977) have given considerable weight to both conceptual and empirical problems in scientific progress. For Laudan, progress consisted of achieving a balance between empirical advances and conceptual dilemmas; scientific progress was, in fact, viewed as the resolution of problems through developments based on "fact," without the addition of new conceptual troubles. Toulmin (1972) also emphasized the important role of concepts in the quest for knowledge, and gave them such prominence that he devoted an entire volume of his work to a discussion of progress and the maintenance of continuity in a discipline, specifically through conceptual change and development. Thus, by improving or otherwise developing concepts, a discipline could make considerable advancements in achieving its intellectual goals (Toulmin, 1972).

Although these philosophers, and a vast array of other scholars, have placed a considerable emphasis on concept development, we tend to know much more about how to tackle empirical concerns than we do about means to resolve conceptual barriers to progress. As a result there has been a substantial gap in the literature concerning concept development and, consequently, in scientific activity as well. This book is an attempt to fill that gap. Actually, no single text could ever fill such a chasm, nor do the contents of this book exhaust the domain of knowledge that concerns concepts and concept development. Nevertheless, we do hope to call attention to conceptual problems and provide a basis for systematic and rigorous inquiry to address them. It is our wish to encourage additional work to develop new methods or to expand on the ones presented here.

The appropriate use of concept development techniques is not always clear. In some instances, certain features of an area of inquiry may be prominent and point to the need for such methods. Most common, perhaps, is a researcher's desire to operationalize or, at least, clarify a concept as a preliminary step in a formal investigation. However, we would argue that in many situations problems confronted in nursing knowledge may be primarily, if not strictly, conceptual in nature. Some of the more obvious conceptual problems include vague terminology, ambiguity regarding the definitions of important concepts in nursing, and inconsistencies among theories. For example, concepts such as self-care and coping are used often in nursing and are generally considered to be important. However, they also are defined and used in widely varying ways. This variation is both confusing and retards scientific advancement in these areas.

Concept development methods also may be appropriate in some less obvious instances: the classification of nursing phenomena, the need for new ways to address or describe a situation in nursing, or the synthesis of existing knowledge concerning a concept of interest. Sometimes concept development methods can be helpful to answer what-is-going-on-here type questions (for example, is a particular client experiencing grief?), and perhaps even some ethical problems can be illuminated by such techniques. For example, consider the new dimensions that might be added to discussions concerning the termination of life support in cases of persistent vegetative states if there were systematic effort to identify various conceptions of "personhood" (Cowles, 1984). What constitutes personhood, as just one example, lies at the base of many ethical problems. It is not a question that can be answered empirically, but lends itself well to concept development techniques.

Fortunately, work on conceptual problems seems to have been increasing in recent years. Yet it still tends to be limited in terms of scope, depth, and methods. Concept development generally has been limited to the obviously abstract and is focused most often on concept analysis, especially adaptations of Wilson's (1963) work. While such studies continue to make a significant contribution to nursing knowledge development, they fail to address the broad range of problems, methods, and issues relevant to this type of inquiry. In short, the full potential of concept analysis, as well as other means to develop concepts, has yet to be tapped by nurse scholars.

Continuing and perhaps escalating the current pace of progress in nursing knowledge requires work on both the empirical and the conceptual matters that confront clinicians, educators, and reseachers in nursing. We do not intend that this statement be misconstrued as yet another contribution to existing methods debates. The arguments about qualitative and quantitative research, a recent focus of methodological debate (Duffy, 1985; Goodwin & Goodwin, 1984; Moccia, 1988), are tiresome enough (and, at this point in nursing's development, frequently superficial) without our giving the impression of taking sides. Besides, the variety of concept development techniques, if taken as a separate class of methods, do not necessarily fit clearly within just one of these categorizations. Nor do we want to confuse the matter further by introducing a third category of research into the discussion. Instead, researchers need to be driven by the questions they pose or by the specific problem for which a solution is sought. Thus, we call attention to some different types of problems that may have received inadequate attention in the past, and provide a few means to address them with quality inquiry.

As mentioned previously, the discussions and methods presented in this text do not exhaust the body of knowledge on concept development. We believe, however, that they are representative of the state of this art. In compiling this collection we sought both well-established and less-developed approaches to concept development. Thus, this text contains a blend of tried-and-true methods, along with more recent, innovative strategies.

In addition to the many other aims of this book, we also hoped to achieve balance in the discussions included. Doing so, however, proved to be a difficult task. Some of the methods presented are more complex, have a longer history, or are more developed than others. In such cases, the authors simply had more to contribute in discussing these approaches. Others could be described only in less complex or less specific ways by virtue of their state of development. Consequently, some discussions of methods are accompanied by example chapters to illustrate not only the results of completed research but the detailed procedures involved in a study using that particular method.

Equal treatment of approaches, then, could not be achieved relative to length or depth of discussion. Instead, the goal was to achieve a balanced overview of the various types and applications of methods available, and to balance the philosophical, methodological, and practical aspects of concept development as a whole. The book begins with a sort of intellectual history of the subject of concepts, focusing on the philosophical aspects and foundations of concepts and concept development. This chapter addresses our belief that the *how* of something (that is, the methods of concept development) must be associated with knowledge of *why* (the rationale) and what it *means* to use such methods. Knafl and Deatrick then present an overview of various techniques to provide a comparison and contrast as a basis for increasing understanding and decision making regarding the primary methods that follow. Where appropriate, the major works are followed by an actual example of the method described for additional clarity.

Following these discussions is a section in which we captured some less-well-known or newer (or both) ideas and some unique applications. Haase and her associates' discussion of the simultaneous concept analysis procedure presents an innovative application of concept analysis to clarify a range of related concepts. Broome's discussion addresses the contributions to concept development that are made with an integrated literature review. The continuing interest in nursing diagnosis and the recent attention to the need for systematic inquiry—such as concept development techniques— to develop diagnostic statements prompted the inclusion of a chapter addressing this specific area of nursing concern.

We conclude this text with additional discussion of the applications of concept development techniques. This reflects our belief that not only is concept development pursued too infrequently (for whatever reason), but also that the vast range of productive uses of such methods may not be recognized. Although concluding chapters in books often are used to bring closure to the text, we hope that this final chapter will open doors to increased recognition, use, and expansion of concept development techniques. Such an occurrence can only provide fuel for progress, whether through increasing awareness and discussion or—what would be the best outcome—by providing workable solutions to some perplexing and very real conceptual problems in nursing.

REFERENCES

Cowles, K. V. (1984). Life, death, and personhood. *Nursing Outlook, 32,* 169–172.
Duffy, M. E. (1985). Designing nursing research: The qualitative-quantitative debate. *Journal of Advanced Nursing, 10,* 225–232.
Goodwin, L. D., & Goodwin, W. L. (1984). Qualitative vs. quantitative research or qualitative and quantitative research? *Nursing Research, 33,* 378—380.
Laudan, L. (1977). *Progress and its problems.* Berkeley, Calif: University of California Press.
Moccia, P. (1988). A critique of compromise: Beyond the methods debate. *Advances in Nursing Science, 10*(4), 1–9.
Toulmin, S. (1972). *Human understanding.* Princeton: Princeton University Press.
Wilson, J. (1963). *Thinking with concepts.* London: Cambridge University Press.

Chapter 2

Philosophical Foundations of Concept Development

BETH L. RODGERS

*O*ne of the most important issues facing researchers and others who desire to use or at least understand concept development concerns the philosophical foundations and assumptions associated with the various methods. This philosophical background has a tremendous influence on decisions concerning the design of a study, the interpretation of findings, and the eventual application of results. Unfortunately, although the development of concepts generally is considered to be a significant activity in the expansion of nursing knowledge, relatively little attention has been directed toward uncovering the philosophical issues associated with concepts and existing techniques for concept analysis and development.

I first became aware of the many philosophical issues associated with concept development when I began to search for means to resolve the conceptual problems that are abundant in nursing. Significant and valuable empirical research had been done to address many critical problems of interest in nursing; yet conceptual problems continued to plague efforts to develop nursing's knowledge base. As I learned more about nursing and knowledge development, it became increasingly evident that difficulties associated with vague and ambiguous terminology, definitions of crucial concepts, theoretical inconsistencies, and at times what seemed to be mass confusion about ideas fundamental to nursing knowledge and practice presented great barriers to progress in nursing.

Inquiry oriented toward resolving conceptual problems would be a major step in providing a solid foundation for continuing knowledge development. Contemporary philosophers provided an impetus for such work by pointing out that knowledge development and, consequently, progress are not dependent solely on empirical inquiry but require attention to conceptual concerns and growth as well (Laudan, 1977; Toulmin, 1972). It was not clear, however, what means or methods and, especially, what philosophical rationale would support work to address such problems.

I began searching for methods and a philosophical basis appropriate to attack such problems and to explore concept analysis as a potentially viable method. Concept analysis was a relatively well-recognized method for resolving some of the types of conceptual problems I had identified throughout my career in nursing (Chinn & Jacobs, 1987; Chinn & Kramer, 1991; Walker & Avant, 1988; Wilson, 1963) and one that lent itself well to some important concerns in nursing (Boyd, 1985; Duffy, 1987; Forsyth, 1980; Gibson, 1991; Knafl & Deatrick, 1986; Matteson & Hawkins, 1990; Meize-Grochowski, 1984; Rawnsley, 1980; Rew, 1986; Simmons, 1989). However, it was difficult and perhaps even naive as a researcher to merely accept such methods as legitimate or necessarily effective. It was important (so I was told) to understand the algebraic derivations of the statistical forms of analysis that I had studied. Similarly, I wanted to understand the philosophical derivations of methods oriented toward concept analysis and development.

The basic structure of the available methods indicated that some important assumptions were being made, yet it was not clear exactly what these assumptions were or whether they were reasonable or defensible. The overriding question became what does it *mean* to use these methods, along with the related query, what will I have when I finish the study? Specifically, to use these methods appropriately, there was a need to know not only that they would work but how they worked, and to validate my own assumption that clarification or development of a concept would, indeed, make a contribution to nursing knowledge.

In an effort to answer these questions I found volumes of literature on the subject of concepts, spread throughout several disciplines, with a consensus that there is an important relationship between concepts and knowledge. But I also found overwhelming debates regarding the nature of concepts, their roles in the development of knowledge, and a variety of implications for concept analysis and development. The notion of *concepts* had been the focus of much discussion and, perhaps, even abuse. It was easy to agree with Toulmin's (1972) poignant observation that "the term 'concept' is in danger becoming [sic] an irredeemably vague catch-all . . . it already carries as much intellectual load as it can safely bear and possibly more" (pp. 8–9). The fundamental question that had to be answered before proceeding with any attempt at concept development remained: What is a concept?

Nearly every writer who addresses the subject of knowledge must at some point grapple with the question of concepts—what they are, what roles they have, and how they relate to the development of knowledge. The mere volume of literature available on the subject makes it unreasonable, if not impossible, to accomplish an exhaustive review of existing thought regarding concepts and concept development. Nevertheless, it is possible to gain insight into predominant issues by exploring the major philosophical schools of thought and the writings of the prominent individuals who represent these diverse viewpoints.

Before beginning such a review, it is important to note that discussions relevant to concept development in nursing are not limited to the writings of philosophers and nurse scholars. The field of psychology in particular has offered a great many insights on the subject. A large volume of work in this discipline has been directed toward discussions of how an individual acquires or forms certain concepts and carries out acts of categorization, a primary function of concepts. Consequently, examples from this body of research are included in this chapter where appropriate as they provide additional clarification and, especially, empirical evidence in reference to major philosophical viewpoints. Such work is important in an attempt to understand the nature of concepts in general; although it is relevant to note that the views presented in psychology are quite similar to, and are derived from, the major trends found in philosophy.

Nursing Views of Concepts

A phrase familiar to anyone who has explored concepts, theories, and existing frameworks in nursing is that concepts are the "building blocks of theory." When the focus becomes more specific, however, the views of *concepts* presented by nurse authors reflect the diversity of approaches to this topic.

CONCEPTS AND EMPIRICAL REALITY

Some authors have focused primarily on the relationship between concepts and empirical or observable reality, arguing that concepts are essentially symbolic of objective elements in the world (Kim, 1983; Walker & Avant, 1983, 1988). Jacox (1974), for example, indicated that "words that describe objects, properties, events, and relations among these are called descriptive terms or concepts," and pointed out that "a major task in the definition of concepts is to specify the part of the empirical world that they are intended to represent" (p. 5). Similarly, Hardy (1974) defined *concepts* as "labels, categories, or selected properties of objects to be studied ... concepts are the dimensions, aspects, or attributes of reality which interest the scientist" (p. 100). Becker (1983) also emphasized observation, and indicated that "concepts arise in the mind of an individual as a result of attempts to make order out of that which is observed" (p. 53). Also characteristic of such views of concepts was the definition provided by Keck (1986), in which concepts were referred to as "the subject matter of theory. They are symbolic representations of the things or events of which phenomena are composed. Concepts represent some aspect of reality that can be quantified" (p. 16). These views all have in common an emphasis on the external or observed world in reference to the formation and nature of concepts.

CONCEPTS AND COGNITION

Other nurse authors have discussed concepts with an emphasis on the mind and human thought (King, 1988), a view exemplified by Watson's (1979) definition of a *concept* as "a mental picture or a mental image, a word that symbolizes ideas and meanings and expresses an abstraction" (pp. 61–62). Meleis (1985) also focused on cognition in her discussion of concepts. According to this author,

> *Concepts evolve out of a complex constellation of impressions, per-*
> *ceptions, and experiences ... concepts are a mental image of reality*
> *tinted with the theorist's perception, experience, and philosophical bent.*
> *They function as a reservoir and an organizational entity and bring*
> *order to observations and perceptions. They help to flag related ideas*
> *and perceptions without going into detailed descriptions. (p. 127)*

Unlike other cognitively oriented definitions, Meleis gave particular emphasis to the role of individual perception in the formation of concepts.

CONCEPTS AND LANGUAGE

A few authors have addressed concepts in reference to language, specifically relating a concept to a particular word. Diers (1979), for example, described a concept as "simply a word to which meaning has been attached through formal definition or common usage" (p. 69). Similarly, Tadd & Chadwick (1989) defined a concept as "the meaning of a word" (p. 156). Occasionally *concept* is defined in regard to a general social aspect. Duldt and Giffin (1985), for example, noted that a concept is a "timeless, abstract, impersonal idea that serves as a norm" (p. 95), and thus pointed out, along with Diers, the possibility that concepts are shared or learned. Since language is essentially social in nature, these authors indicated that personal interaction may be a significant factor in the formation or development of concepts, a view that was noticeably absent in other discussions of concepts.

It is obvious from all these examples that there are numerous ways to approach the subject of concepts. The diversity of views expressed by these nurse authors raises questions about concepts in regard to the processes of human thought, the relationship between concepts and empirical reality and between concepts and language, and the role of social contexts in reference to concept development. An examination of major writings in philosophy provides insight into the generation and implications of such views for knowledge development in nursing.

Philosophical Views of Concepts

The diversity of definitions for the term *concept* presented by nurse authors essentially parallel the variety of viewpoints found in the literature of philosophy. Long-standing debates, focused on the nature and forms of concepts and the role of concepts in the development of knowledge, have resulted in the emergence of two principal philosophical schools of thought. These views are commonly referred to as the entity and dispositional theories of concepts.

ENTITY THEORIES OF CONCEPTS

Entity theories of concepts are characterized by their primary emphasis on concepts as specific things or entities. Typically, concepts are discussed as universal essences (Aristotle, 1947, 1984), abstract ideas in the mind (Descartes, 1644/1960; Kant, 1781/1965; Locke, 1690/1975), or words and their meanings (Frege, 1952a, 1952b; Wittgenstein, 1921/1981). These entities generally are considered to correspond with, or to match directly, actual elements of reality. For example, according to such views the concept of health should correspond with some real and objective "thing," whether abstract or concrete, commonly referred to using the term *health*. Entity theories dominate much of the early literature in philosophy in some form; they still can be found in current writings as some of the examples from nursing indicate.

Dispositional theories, in contrast, present concepts as habits or capacities for certain behaviors. Characteristic behaviors include the ability to use language effectively and the performance of specific mental or physical acts. For example, according to a dispositional viewpoint, a nurse could perform a technique aseptically only when the individual nurse has a grasp of the concept of asepsis. Similarly, acting in a professional manner is dependent upon the individual nurse's concept of professional. Consequently, while entity theories focus specifically on the concept itself as a "thing," dispositional theories emphasize the use of concepts and the behaviors that they make possible. Examples of dispositional theories are rarely found in a pure form in philosophy. However, British philosopher Ryle (1949, 1971a, 1971b, 1971c) and the later writings of Wittgenstein (1953/1968) made significant contributions to the overall development of such views.

Although entity and dispositional theories of concepts are considerably different, there is no formal line of division between the two schools of thought. Philosophers, as well as nurses and others who write on the subject, are not easily categorized as clear advocates of one approach or the other. Often, there are considerable areas of overlap, and characterization of a particular viewpoint can be based only on the author's primary emphasis.

It is important to note as well that if the development of views of concepts in philosophy is examined over time, there initially appears to be a smooth chronological progression. Certainly, philosophical thinking does exhibit some trends, but the transitions that have occurred throughout history do not necessarily demonstrate fluid shifts in thought. Exploration of the variety of viewpoints concerning what a concept is demonstrates the complex history of the subject and the influences that philosophical foundations have on current applications of concept development in nursing.

Concepts and Essentialism. One of the more familiar approaches to concept development is the method of concept analysis that is used to "define" existing concepts (Chinn & Jacobs, 1987; Rodgers, 1989a; Walker & Avant, 1988; Wilson, 1963). The roots for this approach are traced easily to the writings of Aristotle in the fourth century, B.C., and the subsequent development of what is commonly known as the classical approach to analysis. Aristotle (1947) pointed out that the purpose of scientific inquiry was to identify or demonstrate the "essence" of things, in other words, the attributes fundamental to their individual natures and that set each thing apart from all others. According to Aristotle (1947, 1984), the essences determined through analysis were "true universals"; they were thought to exist on a level removed from actual concrete objects and, consequently, to be unaffected by change and motion in the world.

In an approach typical of an entity theory, Aristotle described these concepts or essences as the special "objects" associated with thinking, and argued that they were formed in the mind through a process referred to as "successive generalization." In successive generalization, the mind moves from individual or particular objects or events to progressively broader categories of similar objects or events, focusing on the characteristics common to all classes. As Aristotle described it, this process eventually leads to the identification of essences or attributes that apply universally to entire classes of objects and thus provides a means to categorize various aspects of reality. Concepts, then, represent the essence of certain classes and are universally true of all members of a class. This idea becomes clearer when it is viewed in reference to Aristotle's extensive background in biological studies and his interest in the development of taxonomies to definitively categorize various classes of biological species based on the essential features of each class.

It is easy to see how this view contributed to subsequent developments in understanding concepts and methods of concept development, particularly concept analysis as it is currently represented in nursing. First, Aristotle established the process of definition as a fundamental scientific activity, and thus legitimized efforts to analyze and define concepts. In addition, he provided a foundation for methods of analysis by demonstrating that concepts are abstractions, comprised of the essential and unchanging features of elements or objects in the world. Ideas related to this view of essentialism emerged with new strength in the early twentieth century. However, the emphasis on concepts as special entities themselves, the objects of thought, gained a considerable following long before that time.

Concepts as Ideas

René Descartes. Entity theories particularly began to flourish in the mid-seventeenth century. Much of the stimulus for the further development of entity theories during that time can be attributed to Descartes (1644/1960). Particularly significant was Descartes's argument that the mind (soul) and body (physical reality) are distinctly different substances (the infamous Cartesian "dualism"). Descartes did not argue that the mind and body are totally separate; in fact, Descartes was careful to point out that they were intricately connected (by the pineal gland, according to Descartes). The dualism arose from his position that the mind and the body each had unique features that distinguished these two aspects of existence. The distinguishing feature for bodies was that they were "extended"; in other words, they occupied space in physical reality. The mind, in contrast, was referred to as the "unextended thinking substance," which formed the essence of human nature. According to Descartes, the central feature of the mind was the distinct group of entities referred to as "ideas," which comprised the focus of all cognitive processes. Knowledge consisted essentially of ideas so "clear and distinct" that they were beyond any possibility of doubt.

Descartes subsequently established his rationalist method of inquiry, based on the notion of doubt, as a means to develop knowledge, particularly to distinguish knowledge from belief and opinion. Although this method had little direct bearing on concept development techniques as they are currently utilized, Descartes' emphasis on "clear and distinct" may have provided some incentive for later philosophers who also emphasized rigid clarity in regard to individual concepts. Most significant, however, was his dualism of the mind and body, which led later philosophers to focus their own arguments concerning concepts on one of the two identified aspects of human existence—on either the inner, mental realm or the outer, physical world.

John Locke. Locke (1690/1975) pursued the emphasis on *inner* reality (ideas and the mind) in his discussion of concepts in the *Essay Concerning Human Understanding.* Locke defined an idea as "the object of understanding when a man [sic] thinks ... whatever it is, which the mind can be employed about in thinking" (1690/1975, p. 47). However, in contrast to Descartes's position that ideas could be innate, acquired prior to any experience, Locke argued that ideas were derived exclusively from experience. According to Locke, experience consisted of observation of either the external world (sensation) or of the internal operations of the mind (reflection). Through experience the mind was passively presented with simple ideas with each representing "nothing but *one uniform appearance*" (p. 119), or one particular or individual aspect of reality. From these simple ideas, the mind created generalizations, through a process referred to as "*abstraction,*" that is, "ideas taken from particular beings become general representatives of all of the same kind" (p. 159). In other words, Locke argued that the mind discerned among ideas, categorized similar things, and thereby formed "complex ideas." As abstractions from the particulars encountered in reality, these categories of complex ideas assumed a relatively universal character and formed the basis for human knowledge. Actual knowledge, according to Locke, was "nothing but the perception of the connexion and agreement or disagreement and repugnancy of any of our ideas" (p. 525), a process that ultimately included the comparison and sorting of ideas to establish a consistent and coherent body of knowledge.

The active role taken by the mind in the formation of complex ideas led to the possibility that concepts could vary from one mind to the next, or become unclear or confused. Interestingly, Locke (1690/1975) related such occurrences to problems in individual thought processes (pp. 161–163). Obscure or confused ideas, according to Locke, resulted from either dull sensory organs or the inappropriate combination of simple ideas to form the more complex ones (concepts). Similarly, Locke argued that in some instances there may be a confused connection of a name or word symbol with an idea, which led to difficulties in attempts to communicate or share concepts. However, Locke generally emphasized that the ideas and the associated cognitive processes were at fault when problems existed with ambiguous or unclear concepts.

For Locke, then, as for Descartes, concepts were ideas in some form and served as the objects of human thought. According to these philosophers, concepts were inherently private entities in that they resided exclusively in the individual mind. Locke did address the possibility that concepts could be communicated with other persons, but this could be accomplished only through a complex system of signs or symbols. Analysis, clarification, and development of concepts as mental entities presumably could be accomplished only by gaining direct access to an individual's mind. Consequently, in these views, concepts were not amenable to any techniques currently used for purposes of concept development. The only improvement or clarification of concepts that could be accomplished had to be focused on individual processes of thought and idea formation. In addition, Locke's argument that all ideas were derived from experience suggested a direct relationship between an idea and a sensory or reflective experience. Therefore, an understanding of a concept required not only insight into actual thought processes but examination of correspondence between an idea or concept and the experience that produced it.

Immanuel Kant. Kant (1781/1965) also focused on concepts as ideas but, unlike Locke, did not view them as the result of experience. Instead, Kant argued that concepts existed in the mind even before any experience and, in fact, actually made experience possible. Knowledge, according to

Kant, resulted in part from the combination of experience with the pre-existing content and capabilities of the human mind. Concepts provided the rules necessary for this essential process of combination.

Unlike earlier views, Kant (1781/1965) denied that concepts had any direct relationship with objective reality and similarly rejected the notion that the definition of a concept revealed the essence of any associated object. However, Kant did address the possibility of defining concepts as a means to provide clarification, although he identified limitations as to the types of concepts that could be defined. A priori concepts, those that existed in the mind before experience, could not be defined since, according to Kant, gaining a complete definition of such a concept simply could not be accomplished; definition on this level "really only means to present the complete, original concept of a thing" (p. 586). Empirical concepts similarly "[could not] be defined at all but only *made explicit*" (p. 586). Only concepts that had been "arbitrarily invented" were amenable to any attempt at definition or clarification.

Conclusion. These prominent philosophers—Descartes, Locke, and Kant—made a tremendous contribution to current discussions of concepts. They postulated various ways in which concepts were acquired, the possibility that vague or ambiguous concepts impeded the development of knowledge, and the variety of types or levels of concepts that existed. Most significant, perhaps, was that they drew considerable attention to the importance of concepts in discussions about knowledge in general, even though there was tremendous diversity in their individual approaches to concepts and related epistemological questions.

In spite of the differences in their views, all three philosophers relied heavily on the notion of *ideas* and an emphasis on the inner workings of the human mind. This focus presented problems in regard to the means by which concepts could be clarified or further developed. As noted previously, the emphasis on concepts as exclusively mental entities placed concepts in a realm where they were not accessible as a focus for inquiry. Locke did argue that concepts might be symbolized through words for purposes of communication, possibly providing some means for analysis or development. However, this position served only to raise questions about the connection between concepts, specific words, and other acts used to express individual thoughts. Some philosophers, most notably Frege (1952a, 1952b), reacted very negatively to such discussions of concepts, and referred to them as "psychologism" in reference to the belief that the meaning of words could be attributed only to specific mental processes. The result was a shift in the focus of discussions of concepts from the mind to external reality, a development undoubtedly fueled by demonstrated advances in the natural sciences and the earlier acceptance of positivism in discussions of scientific knowledge (Ayer, 1959; Silva & Rothbart, 1983; Webster, Jacox, & Baldwin, 1981).

Concepts and Logic. Frege (1952a, 1952b) offered what might be considered a "realist" revolt against the early mental and psychological focus in discussions of concepts and knowledge. As with many of his predecessors, Frege (1952b) acknowledged the importance of concepts in the development of knowledge. He also recognized the existence of a great deal of confusion regarding the term, noting that "the word 'concept' is used in various ways; its sense is sometimes psychological, sometimes logical, and sometimes perhaps a confused mixture of both" (1952b, p. 42). For his own views, Frege adopted principles of logic as they applied to language, and focused specifically on the distinction between concepts and objects as revealed through specific parts of language.

The connection between concepts and objects had been confused somewhat in earlier discussions of concepts in which philosophers argued that concepts arose directly from experience with specific objects (Locke, 1690/1975) or that they made experience possible (Kant, 1781/1965). Difficulties were encountered primarily in attempts to differentiate clearly between a concept and its corresponding object. Frege attempted to resolve the confusion about concepts and objects through attention to their corresponding terms or denotative expressions. Frege identified two primary categories of words: proper names and predicates. Proper names were said to include terms such as *blue* and *two,* which were thought to represent specific objects. Concepts, in contrast, were viewed as predicates; "[a concept] is, in fact, the reference of a grammatical predicate" (1952b, p. 43). Concepts, therefore, represent the "existence of a property" (p. 48) and, as such, are entities that are true for some objects and false for others.

Admittedly, the term *two* seems an unlikely example of a proper name to designate an object. However, a closer examination of Frege's view of language helps to clarify his point. A concept, as expressed by a grammatical predicate, was represented in language by an incomplete statement, which became a complete sentence by the addition of a proper name. In the statement "two is a prime number," *two* was a proper name and designated an object according to Frege. The remainder of the statement, "is a prime number," was incomplete and required the addition of the *name* of an object to make any sense grammatically. As the predicate in this statement, *prime number* represented a characteristic or property of *two* and thus denoted a concept.

For a concept to be predicated of an object appropriately, in other words, to present a characteristic of the object, Frege (1952a) argued that the concept had to be extremely clear. As he pointed out:

> *A definition of a concept (of a possible predicate) must be complete; it must unambiguously determine, as regards any object, whether or*

not it falls under the concept . . . the concept must have a sharp bound-
ary . . . a concept that is not sharply defined is wrongly termed a concept.
(p. 159)

Without an absolutely clear concept of *prime number* it would be impossible to determine whether or not the concept was appropriately predicated
of the object known as *two*. Frege thus characterized concepts in regard
to their linguistic denotations as grammatical predicates. In addition, he
pointed out that concepts must have rigid boundaries, with the domain of
the concept expressed as a set of necessary and sufficient conditions—the
critical conditions or attributes necessary to define the concept and that
were by themselves sufficient to distinguish it clearly from all other concepts.

Frege's position regarding the boundaries and clarity of concepts indicated that concepts have an essence that is unchanging over time and across
contexts. The requirement that the boundaries of each concept be clearly
delineated emphasized the static nature of concepts and the belief that any
single concept could be viewed in isolation, not only apart from its context,
but without regard to its relationship with other concepts. The ultimate
goal, it seemed, was to generate concepts that were so clearly delineated
that the concepts could, indeed, be determined true or false in reference
to any situation or object that was confronted. For example, either *two* is
a prime number or it is not, and this determination could be evaluated as
true or false only if the concept was precise and exceptionally clear.

The Search for an Ideal Language. The impact of Frege's realist approach to concepts was evident throughout the early twentieth century.
The emphasis on language, a particularly significant aspect of Frege's works,
provided a considerable basis for the writings of Wittgenstein, another prominent German philospher. Wittgenstein's works can be divided into two
periods, with radically different views expressed during each stage in the
development of his thought. During his early period, Wittgenstein (1921/
1981) produced his famous text, the *Tractatus Logico-philosophicus.* In
discussing the importance of this work, Hartnack (1965) indicated that "the
Tractatus is a book of just over eighty pages, but it has exercised a greater
influence on twentieth-century philosophy than almost any other single
work" (p. 45). This work provided a particularly great stimulus for members
of the Vienna Circle, a group generally synonymous with the Logical Positivism movement (Ayer, 1959; Carnap, 1956; Russell, 1914; Schlick, 1959).

The influence of Frege was evident in the *Tractatus* and in the notebooks
Wittgenstein (1979) left behind, which showed the painstaking development of his ideas. However, Wittgenstein differed from Frege somewhat in
his views of language and concepts. Frege regarded language as a system
of symbols that clearly represented concepts; Wittgenstein, in contrast,
discussed language in general as a system that directly corresponded to

physical reality. According to Wittgenstein (1921/1981), words symbolized actual objects, not mental images or thoughts. Wittgenstein agreed that there was a close relationship between concepts and language, but devoted very little attention to a specific discussion of concepts. Instead, he considered language itself to be the primary concern, and focused on language as a "picture" of reality, complete with rules for determining correspondence between language and reality (Wittgenstein, 1921/1981). In fact, Wittgenstein and the members of the Vienna Circle devoted considerable attention to the notion of constructing an "ideal language" that would mirror precisely the structure of the external world. Such a language was presumed to eliminate all ambiguity and enable the construction of statements that provided a picture of how reality really is. It was an ambitious goal, to say the least, but by virtue of the many problems raised by such a language not a very realistic or even appropriate focus.

Contributions and Problems with Entity Theories. All the views previously addressed are representative of the entity theory of concepts. Such theories have dominated much of philosophical thought on the subject of concepts. Certainly, the contributions of philosophers associated with this general approach to concepts cannot be underestimated. There is little disagreement, for example, that concepts are mental or cognitive in nature. In addition, entity views provide the impetus and rationale for the clarification of concepts, establishing it as a legitimate form of inquiry and providing numerous insights into methodological concerns.

However, as with any philosophical position, there are numerous problems associated with such views. One particularly glaring difficulty is related to Descartes's dualism, which contributed to philosophers' emphasizing either internal thought processes or external reality in their discussions of concepts. Toulmin (1972) poignantly noted that this background contributed to "intractable conundrums about the relations between the 'inner' and 'outer,' or private and public, aspects of mental life" (p. 197). Language provided one means to establish a connection between the public and private realms of existence, revealing how inner thoughts might be exposed to public scrutiny. However, the particular way in which philosophers such as Locke, Frege, and Wittgenstein discussed language only served to generate confusion about the precise connection between concepts and words. In fact, according to such views, especially those of Frege and Wittgenstein, the development of a concept was easily viewed in terms of clarification of a specific word, its reference, and the further development of language in general. Individual thoughts or *ideas* had little role in this process of knowledge development.

The emphasis on correspondence, whether between words and concepts, words and objects, or concepts and objects (or experience) is undoubtedly one of the most troublesome aspects of prominent entity views and one of the "intractable conundrums." The term *health,* as just one example, is easily used to point out some of the difficulties with these views. Undoubtedly, the word *health* conjures considerably different images or concepts for different people, relative to culture, socioeconomic status, personal experience, and a variety of other factors. Health may be conceptualized as the absence of disease (another troublesome concept), in reference to individual functioning and independence, or in any number of diverse ways. It is clear that the concept typically expressed using the term *health* is not the same for all people.

Similarly, none of the possible conceptualizations of health necessarily corresponds with any real object. On a highly abstract level, there may be some object to which health (or hope, pain, or grief, as a few other examples) corresponds. There also may be certain empirical correlates, evaluated using accepted measurement tools, that help to determine the presence or absence of health. However, conceptualization of human experiences, such as health, cannot be accomplished definitively on the basis of measurement devices alone, which are not without error themselves. Consequently, the requirement for correspondence on any level and the determination of *truth* versus *falsity* in regard to concepts is both philosophically troublesome and inconsistent with everyday existence.

In support of this criticism are studies conducted in the field of psychology that have shown a severe discrepancy between the positions advocated by entity views and actual human processes of conceptualization (Armstrong, Gleitman, & Gleitman, 1983; Fehr, 1988; McCloskey & Glucksberg, 1978; Medin & Schaffer, 1978). First, studies have shown that, for many concepts, even experts in a field may be unable to specify the conditions necessary and sufficient (or essential) in regard to a particular concept (Medin, 1989). Second, the classical theory of thinking, as such entity views often are called, implies that no one example of a concept is any better than another; all examples must possess the same core of essential attributes. Undoubtedly, it is possible to assemble a diverse group of people, all of whom might possess whatever are considered to be the essential attributes of health; yet some of these individuals certainly would be judged as more typical of the concept than others. As noted previously, the judgment of the "best" examples of the concept of health could vary with the personal characteristics of the judge. It is possible to argue that some of the judges would be false in their conceptualizations based on a strict interpretation of the notion of necessary and sufficient conditions. This view, however, would require that individual perceptions be ignored. Equally significant, it would be incompatible with actual human practices and how people use the concepts they possess.

Finally, the classical view suggests that it is possible to determine definitively whether a particular instance does, indeed, exemplify a specific concept. Nevertheless, there are numerous examples of situations that are vague in regard to conceptual category membership, such as the determination of whether addictive disorders are "diseases," a recent development that challenged adherents to the popular "germ" interpretation of this concept. Such challenges are not answered by an appeal to the necessary and sufficient conditions of the concept of disease, for these have changed over time and across cultural and even disciplinary contexts.

Entity views, therefore, have presented some philosophical difficulties in discussions of concepts, particularly in regard to the connection between concepts, language, and objects, and reliance on correspondence as the test for the "truth" of a concept. The requirement, imposed by Frege (1952a), that concepts have sharply defined boundaries and the lack of attention to any context in discussions of concepts, raised additional questions. It is debatable whether reality can be so easily partitioned as to make an expectation of infallible distinctions and strict correspondence reasonable (Fehr, 1988). Similarly, the idea that concepts may change over time or across contexts raises concerns about how determinate and clearly delineated concepts can be, as more recent views demonstrate (Rodgers, 1989a, 1989b; Rorty, 1979; Toulmin, 1972; Wittgenstein, 1953/1968). The notion of conceptual change presents a strong case against the call for clear and rigid boundaries, which of necessity cannot vary over time or across contexts.

DISPOSITIONAL THEORIES OF CONCEPTS

Dispositional theories emerged partially in response to the problems with entity views. Interestingly, while it was the interpretation of Wittgenstein's early works (1921/1981, 1979) by logical positivists that provided much of the foundation for the views of concepts that dominated contemporary discussions noted previously, it also was Wittgenstein who provided major criticisms of this approach and contributed to the transition toward dispositional views of concepts. In *Philosophical Investigations* (1953/1968), Wittgenstein denounced the "grave mistakes" (p. vi) contained in his earlier work and drew attention to the *use* of words, rather than the objects to which they referred, as the primary consideration in determining meaning. The rationale for an emphasis on use is clearly presented by Hallett (1967) in his discussion of Wittgenstein's writings:

> *They, objects and shadows [absent facts that are still, nonetheless, thought], are unnecessary for speech. Use is obviously necessary. A word must be used in a certain way if it is to have meaning, if it is to count as speech rather than mere sounds.*
>
> *They are sometimes missing; use never is.*
>
> *Mental pictures are themselves signs; use is not.*
>
> *Mental events are private; use is not . . . whatever the reason for dissatisfaction with object or idea, use always gave satisfaction. (p. 76)*

Consequently, Wittgenstein introduced the idea of language as a "game" to emphasize the aspect of use and to replace the earlier "picture" theory that relied on correspondence for the determination of meaning.

Wittgenstein's (1953/1968) discussion of "language games" called attention to the interactive nature of language, where "one party calls out the words, the other acts on them" (1953/1968, p. 5). A language game, therefore, is comprised of language and the actions associated with its use. Unlike the picture theory, which advocated strict correspondence, language games act as "objects of comparison"; clarity could be provided through identification of similar and dissimilar features of various language acts. As such, a language game serves as a "measuring-rod; not as a preconceived idea to which reality *must* correspond" (pp. 50–51). It provides a standard or a guide, not an absolute determinant of truth or falsehood.

Wittgenstein (1953/1968) referred to his new position as the principle of "family resemblances." In other words, the term *health* could reasonably be used to describe diverse individuals because each person sufficiently resembled the concept of health and displayed characteristics that resembled health, not because the individual possessed a finite core of essential attributes. According to this later view, it was not reasonable to expect perfectly clear "pictures" of all concepts, particularly those that pertained to aesthetics or ethics (p. 36). In a direct refutation of Frege's earlier position that a concept with a blurred edge is not really a concept, Wittgenstein presented the following questions for consideration:

Is an indistinct photograph a picture of a person at all?

Is it even always an advantage to replace an indistinct picture by a sharp one? Isn't the indistinct one often exactly what we need? (p. 34)

Wittgenstein thus rejected the requirements that concepts have rigid and distinct boundaries, that definitions be stated in terms of necessary and sufficient conditions, and that there be a criterion of strict correspondence between concepts and empirical reality.

Instead, Wittgenstein argued that conceptualizations were based upon resemblances or commonalities in the use of a word or concept. According to Wittgenstein (1953/1968), it was the ability to formulate comparisons that provided conceptual clarity. Clarification was to be directed toward "seeing what is common" (p. 34) in the use of a word, not toward uncovering any "essence." Appropriately, psychologists often refer to such a position as the "fuzzy set" theory, where "category membership [the applicability of a concept] is a matter of degree rather than all or none" (McCloskey & Glucksberg, 1978, p. 462).

The emphasis on the use of concepts was a prominent feature of Wittgenstein's *Philosophical Investigations* and set this work apart from many of the earlier contributions to discussions of concepts. Nevertheless, in this text, as in some of his earlier related work (1921/1981, 1979), Wittgenstein was concerned primarily with language. Consequently, the later text is devoted to the development of a complex theoio about language, its struc-ture, and its relationship to reality rather than to a direct exposition of concepts. The views presented in this work are not totally exemplary of dispositional approaches in general, as they lacked sufficient attention to individual capacities or abilities associated with concepts, the distinguishing feature of dispositional theories. It is important to note, however, the tran-sition and the foundation for dispositional views provided by the *Philo-sophical Investigations.*

THE USE OF CONCEPTS

More characteristic of a dispositional theory are the writings of British philosopher Ryle (1949, 1971a, 1971b, 1971c). Like Wittgenstein, Ryle (1971b) rejected the idea that reference to an object is the way to determine the meaning of a concept and adopted the idea of "use" as a central focus in his work. According to Ryle, "the use of an expression, or the concept it expresses, is the role it is employed to perform, not any thing or person or event for which it might be supposed to stand" (1971c, p. 364). Ryle charged philosophy with the task of identifying the criteria governing the logical application of an expression or concept, a task that was to be ac-complished through analytic techniques (1949, p. 329). In other words, through philosophical analysis, Ryle expected that standards or guides could be identified to promote the appropriate use of a concept.

Even for Ryle, concepts were cognitive in nature. Yet, Ryle attempted to overcome the difficulties presented by earlier philosophers who specif-ically emphasized mental processes in discussions of concepts. Refuting the dogma of the mind-body dualism, Ryle argued that there was, indeed, a strong connection between the two aspects of being. References to and, consequently, examination of mental processes could be made in terms of activities that could be witnessed by others:

> *When we describe people as exercising qualities of mind, we are not referring to occult episodes of which their overt acts and utterances are effects; we are referring to those overt acts and utterances themselves. (Ryle, 1949, p. 25)*

Discussions of cognition, therefore, were not necessarily limited to an ex-ploration of the actual processes of thought as they occurred inside the human mind. Rather, cognition could be discussed and even observed through outward, public manifestations. Language served as a particularly important medium for such observations. For Ryle a concept was not the same as a mere word, however; rather, a word or statement served as a means to express individual concepts and therefore was a source of ob-servable evidence of the concepts.

Ryle also suggested that fundamental questions that served as the basis for discussions of concepts be reframed as well. While earlier philosophers asked primarily how concepts (or ideas) were acquired, Ryle (1971c) pointed out that the more appropriate question actually was "what were we unable to do until we had acquired it?" (p. 448). Ryle responded by indicating that the acquisition of a concept enables the management of a range of intellectual and conversational tasks that share features common to the concept. Without the possession or the grasp of a concept, an individual is unable to accomplish or even become involved in such activities.

A concept, then, for Ryle, is an abstracted feature of the world and is integrally related to the ability to perform certain tasks. One of these tasks, and a critical one, is the effective use of language. For Ryle, concepts are neither objects nor the names of objects; they are not inherently true or false, nor are they the components of creating truths or falsehoods. They are, in general, the ability to move effectively through the world. The development of a concept, then, might be viewed as the creation of improved abilities and new ways to function effectively.

Ryle formulated a number of theories of concepts through his writings. Consequently, to say that Ryle strictly equated a concept with a capacity would render an unusually narrow interpretation of this philosopher's contribution to discussions of concepts. What is most significant is Ryle's idea that the use of a word may be an outward manifestation of an individual's grasp of a concept. By providing this insight, Ryle presented a way in which private, mental processes might be accessed and concepts, as mental abstractions, could be analyzed effectively. Individuals move through the world of everyday existence, and the importance of Ryle's works was to point out the role of concepts in that existence. With the influence of Ryle, concepts took on a more pragmatic role, with practical gains to be made through efforts at clarification and development.

Both Ryle and the later Wittgenstein represented significant departures from previous ideas concerning the nature of concepts. Of particular importance was the contrast they offered to earlier views concerning correspondence between concepts and objects and their subsequent emphasis on a public or social aspect of concepts. In psychology the influence of these ideas, particularly Wittgenstein's emphasis on family resemblance, appears in an approach referred to as the "probabilistic" view (Medin, 1989; Smith & Medin, 1981), the "cluster concept" or "prototypical" view, or, as noted previously, the "fuzzy set" theory of concepts (Armstrong et al., 1983; McCloskey & Glucksberg, 1978).

These views represent a substantial improvement over a typical dispositional theory in that the heading *dispositional* is inadequate to capture their uniqueness. Particularly, unlike the positions of Ryle and Wittgenstein, the emphasis in such views goes well beyond the mere use of concepts to their actual nature and their development in the human mind. However, as is the case with a dispositional theory, the primary feature of all these views is that the defining characteristics that comprise a concept are not considered to be "essential" or "necessary and sufficient." Instead, they are regarded only as demonstrating some degree of association with the concept. In a probabilistic view, there is additional concern for the probability with which a characteristic or attribute is associated with a concept. Such views allow for the "typicality" effect, whereby some instances are judged more typical of the concept than others, even though less typical instances still can be characterized using the same concept.

Diagnostic and other taxonomies reflect the probabilistic view in that diagnoses are based on a cluster of presenting characteristics; some characteristics may carry more weight than others. As another example, based on the notion of *family resemblances,* it is possible to describe an individual who has recently experienced the death of a loved one as demonstrating grief and as more typical of grief. Yet, the concept of grief still may be used in reference to individuals who have experienced other types of loss, such as displacement from the home or job. In these latter instances, there is a sufficient resemblance or a reasonable *probability* concerning the defining characteristics of grief and the individual situations, even though they may be viewed as less typical.

In spite of these contributions, several other important concerns about concepts have continued to trouble philosophers and other interested scholars. Some problems were centered around the idea of *use;* Ryle (1971d) devoted an entire paper to a discussion of *use,* yet failed to provide any clear explanation of what *use* really is. In addition, although the Cartesian dualism dissolved somewhat as later philosophers established a relationship between private concepts and public activities such as language, the relationship between concepts and knowledge seemed to be of little interest to such authors. Also of interest, especially to researchers, neither Ryle nor Wittgenstein was a methodologist. Consequently, their writings failed to provide a sufficient foundation for the clarification or development of concepts. As a result, concerns were generated about how their philosophical positions might be translated into methods to enhance the growth of knowledge.

Other concerns about concepts in general warranted attention as well, yet were inadequately addressed by these more recent philosophers. For example, the argument that concepts are at least somewhat public or social in nature raised questions about the role of contextual factors in the use or development of concepts. As Wittgenstein (1953/1968) pointed out, universal categories and concepts intelligible within all cultures can be found only to the extent that there are universal patterns of life and behavior. Since life patterns and behaviors do vary across contexts in many respects, the associated concepts are likely to vary as well. This observation may have methodological implications in efforts to clarify or develop concepts in nursing. Relevant contexts may include cultural and ethnic backgrounds, other social groups, and even disciplinary factors.

In addition to possible variations in concepts across contexts, there is a problem of conceptual change over time. The predominant thought concerning concepts throughout much of history focused on concepts as *universals*, unaffected by change and other forces in the world. This view, which lasted at least through the time of Frege, implored philosophers to "concern themselves with 'concepts' only as timeless, intellectual ideals, towards which the human mind struggles, at best, painfully and little by little" (Toulmin, 1972, p. 56). Such an absolutist tradition disregarded the possibility of historical and social influences having an effect on concepts and the existence of conceptual variation. There can be little doubt, however, that concepts do change. In nursing, perhaps one of the most vivid examples concerns the concept of disease, which has varied widely over time and across a number of distinct cultural and, perhaps, even disciplinary contexts. These dilemmas concerning conceptual variation were addressed rather extensively by Toulmin (1972). Examination of his views provides additional insights in an attempt to understand the diversity of approaches to the discussion of concepts.

THE EVOLUTION OF CONCEPTS

Toulmin (1972) failed to define the term *concept*, but his discussion still added a new dimension to an understanding of this topic. Particularly significant about Toulmin's contribution was his emphasis on the process of conceptual change and the relationship between concepts and scientific progress and development. Following the line of thought that concepts are social in nature, Toulmin (1972) based his argument on this critical assumption:

> *We acquire our grasp of language and conceptual thought... in the course of education and development; and the particular sets of concepts we pick up reflect forms of life and thought, understanding and expression current in our society. (p. 38)*

Toulmin thus considered concepts to be developed through social interaction and a process referred to as "enculturation," which may be accomplished through imitation, simple interaction, or formal education.

Toulmin's work is distinct particularly for this emphasis on the social aspect of concepts. In fact, Toulmin explicitly discussed concepts as the collective possession of a community of concept users, emphasizing the importance of context and socialization in discussions of this topic. Focused specifically on scientific disciplines as the community and context of interest, he also described the relationship between concepts and the advancement of various fields of study.

According to Toulmin (1972), intellectual disciplines are characterized by specific sets of "explanatory ideals"; the "professionals," the human individuals associated with a particular discipline or knowledge base, are driven by certain phenomena that the group desires to explain. Problems were said to result when existing capabilities fell short of reaching these ideals (p. 152). Conceptual problems often accounted for the gap between current understanding and intellectual goals. The development or clarification of concepts, therefore, was viewed as an important component of overall scientific progress.

According to Toulmin, concepts possess "explanatory power" demonstrated by their utility in characterizing phenomena or situations of interest in the discipline. Through a process that entails continuing application of the concept and critical analysis of its contribution to problem solving, the concepts of the science can be altered, refined, or changed altogether, yielding a concept with improved content and explanatory power. According to Toulmin, in any "rational enterprise" concepts survive "because they are still serving their original intellectual functions, or else because they have since acquired other, different functions" (p. 130). Concepts, therefore, are continually changed, or refined, or new concepts are introduced to enhance the problem solving abilities of the discipline. Consequently, the process of concept development occupies a critical role in solving some of the problems relevant to a specific branch of science.

By pointing out the social nature of concepts and the factors and processes associated with concept development and change, Toulmin provided several new possibilities for the conduct of inquiry. First, arguments about the social and contextual (or disciplinary) basis of concepts presented the need for considerations of these aspects in research oriented toward concept development. It may be important for the researcher to consider or work to identify contextual or disciplinary differences associated with particular concepts in the design or conduct of an investigation. The likelihood of conceptual change raises similar concerns and challenges earlier assumptions that a concept may be defined in only one way. Similarly, the notion of essences and rigid and unwavering boundaries for concepts must be reevaluated in light of Toulmin's position and actual examples that demonstrate the existence of conceptual variation and change (Rodgers, 1989a, 1989b).

Toulmin did not specifically address the implications of his views for concept development. However, it is clear in his work that concept development can be of vital importance in the growth of knowledge in a discipline. Particularly, he pointed out the role of concepts in ensuring some continuity and, hence, the identity of a discipline over time and in solving relevant problems within the discipline. The development of concepts, therefore, is seen as a significant research and intellectual activity in the scientific enterprise of nursing. In addition, because concepts have a particular function in a discipline and are viewed as changing and developing over time, it is reasonable, if not desirable, to work toward concepts that are increasingly clear, useful, and effective in problem solving. Recently, Rodgers (1989a, 1989b) has elaborated on and adapted, in part, Toulmin's views to develop an interpretation of concept analysis that shows the implications of conceptual change and the context-dependent nature of concepts for nursing inquiry.

Toulmin's point that concepts exist in the context of scientific disciplines is expanded somewhat in the views of cognitive psychologists who argue for the potential influence of different perspectives in general in regard to concepts. As Medin (1989) pointed out, "something is needed to give concepts life, coherence, and meaning" (p. 1474). This ingredient may be related to the context or theory in which specific exemplars are viewed. In other words, perspectives provided by theories or other contextual bases affect what features are viewed as similar in order to determine the relationship (or resemblance) between certain situations and specific concepts (Medin & Schaffer, 1978). Concepts, therefore, may be not only context-dependent in regard to specific scientific disciplines, as Toulmin (1972) argued, but may evidence even greater variation through the influence of diverse theories. Although Medin (1989) and numerous other psychologists (McCloskey & Glucksberg, 1978) support the importance of similarity (or "family resemblances") in the conceptualization of the situations that humans encounter, theory, existing knowledge, memory (Barsalou & Medin, 1986), and general perspectives (Oden & Lopes, 1982) can affect the use and application of concepts (Rodgers, 1989a, 1989b).

Implications for Concept Development in Nursing

The views presented in the preceding sections reveal the tremendous diversity in attempts to answer questions concerning the nature of concepts, the roles they play, and the relationship between concepts and knowledge. These views undoubtedly raise numerous questions about methodological issues concerning concept development in nursing. Unfortunately, in spite of the tremendous volume of literature on the subject of concepts, there is little specific information available to assist researchers in identifying appropriate designs and procedures for concept development. Even the literature that does include a discussion of methods still leaves the investigator to make many decisions independently.

The current status of knowledge that pertains to concept development precludes the development of specific guidelines and procedures for researchers to follow. In all likelihood there are as many approaches to the development of concepts as there are concepts to be investigated. Nevertheless, there are positions and assumptions that are more defensible and more reasonable in the present context and others that leave the investigation open to greater debate. Although the researcher may have to make independent methodological decisions in many instances, these decisions do not have to be arbitrary ones. Productive use of concept development techniques, therefore, is dependent upon the investigator recognizing the assumptions that underlie the approach employed and the philosophical basis of all methodological decisions. Ultimately, these considerations have a significant impact on the interpretation and utilization of the results of a study.

Selection of a reasonable approach to concept development is contingent upon a variety of factors. First, since concept development always is oriented toward the resolution of some type of conceptual problem, it is important to identify the nature of the problem to be addressed by the research. Laudan (1977) described two major classifications of conceptual problems: (1) "internal" conceptual problems, or problems related to the lack of clarity of basic concepts, and (2) "external" conceptual problems, in which there is a conceptual conflict between competing theories (pp. 49–54). Although Laudan focused on conceptual problems primarily in regard to scientific theories, such problems may appear in numerous different forms for the nurse researcher.

On a practical level, conceptual problems can take a variety of forms: confusing terminology or ambivalent word use to characterize certain situations or phenomena; difficulty synthesizing existing knowledge on a topic, particularly because key concepts have been defined in diverse ways and often arbitrarily; problems defining important concepts for research or theory development; problems or questions concerning the origin of a particular concept and potential change in definition over time; concerns about differences in existing concepts across disciplines that hinder knowledge synthesis, growth, and communication; potential conflicts between concepts and actual situations encountered in nursing; the need for new or more effective concepts to characterize experiences encountered in nursing; and the appropriateness of combining two or more concepts to generate a useful construct. These problems clearly indicate that concept development methods may be appropriate and beneficial in further knowledge development. Different techniques need to be evaluated for their utility in resolving the primary conceptual problem identified by the researcher.

A second concern that needs to be addressed in selecting an approach to concept development involves the nature of concepts in general. In addressing this concern, the researcher can start by identifying his or her general philosophical position regarding concepts. Particularly, the researcher must consider views regarding the rigidity of concepts, the appropriateness of boundaries, the role of social and other contexts in relation to concept definitions and development, and the problem of conceptual change. Positions expressed by Frege (1952a, 1952b), Wittgenstein (1953/ 1968), and Toulmin (1972), noted previously, reveal the diversity of possible responses to these questions. All of these views have considerable implications for methodology and the anticipated outcome of the inquiry.

Similarly, it is necessary to consider the nature of the particular concept of interest. Concepts that are scientific and especially those that have been arbitrarily invented and named for a specific purpose, such as electron or AIDS, may be amenable to more precise definition, particularly when the concept is relatively new and, thus, less likely to have been redefined numerous times. Similarly, such concepts may be evaluated more easily than others in reference to some tangible or measurable aspect of reality. Physiologic concepts are likely to fall into this category; psychosocial concepts, on the other hand, are likely to evidence greater ambiguity, variation, and overlap, and more difficulty in linking them to objective empirical situations.

Concepts that are related to a process (Kim, 1983) present a unique situation as well. Part of the act of defining, clarifying, or otherwise developing concepts often concerns the connection between the concept and specific events or occurrences. Process concepts, however, may not have a clearly identifiable beginning or end point and may be more difficult to clarify in general because of variations that occur at specific points in the process. Clarification of concepts such as grief (Cowles & Rodgers, see Chapter 7) or other concepts that pertain to a process (Westra & Rodgers, 1991) may require special consideration because of the internal variations inherent in the concept.

Another consideration in selecting an approach to concept development concerns the history of the concept. History, in this sense, pertains to the general length of time the concept has been in existence, its estimated time and context of origin, and the translations and adaptations that have occurred over time. Concepts that have been in existence for many decades are likely to have undergone some change and to be applied differently than when initially developed. Although the passing of time theoretically provides the opportunity for further development of a concept, in reality concepts often become more vague and ambiguous over time. In some situations the concept may have been retained in its original form, without attempts to bring about the changes that may have been appropriate as life situations in general changed. The result may be a gross lack of conceptual clarity or a concept that is no longer relevant or effective in application to the situations that are confronted in nursing. Even concepts that are fairly well developed with some consensus about definition may benefit from research to evaluate the applicability of the concept in different settings. Assessment of the current status of knowledge, which may be accomplished through an examination of existing literature, helps to clarify the nature of the conceptual problem and, in turn, helps the researcher determine a productive approach for inquiry.

Methods for concept development offer a significant contribution to expanding the knowledge base of nursing. For these methods to be useful, it is important that the researcher be attentive to the variety of philosophical issues associated with concepts. Particularly, the current status of the concept of interest and the nature of associated conceptual problems need to be considered in selecting appropriate techniques for further development. In addition, the basic assumptions adopted by the investigator have a profound effect on the specific approach to concept development and the interpretation and application of the findings.

In spite of the long history of discussions of concepts and the tremendous diversity of opinion, at present there is only a beginning answer to the question "What is a concept?" There is a consensus that concepts are cognitive in nature and that they are comprised of attributes abstracted from reality, expressed in some form and utilized for some common purpose (Rodgers, 1989b). Consequently, concepts are more than words or mental images alone. In addition, an emphasis on use alone is not sufficient to capture the complex nature of concepts.

There also are substantial empirical data, along with philosophical rationale, to support a family resemblance (cluster concept or fuzzy set) approach to conceptualization. It may be practical, and even desirable, to aim for a high level of clarity and precision in the definition or development of certain concepts. However, this aim does not support an emphasis on entity views with their focus on reduction, necessary and sufficient conditions, rigid boundaries, and context-free interpretations. Instead, in such cases, clarity still must include recognition of the possibility of temporal and contextual change and an appreciation for connections, rather than reduction, to be consistent with current philosophical thought.

Further work is needed to determine whether any position can be universally applicable to all types of concepts, such as "scientific" or "arbitrarily invented" concepts, as they are sometimes called, as compared with more abstract concepts. As philosophers, psychologists, nurses, and other scholars continue to explore the fundamental questions concerning concepts, new answers will emerge and, undoubtedly, new questions as well. At this time it is most important for nurse researchers to recognize the importance of resolving conceptual problems in nursing and to be aware of the philosophical foundations of concept development and their implications for expanding the knowledge base of nursing. A strong and defensible philosophical rationale for decisions made by researchers ultimately is the primary ingredient in efforts to promote conceptual progress in nursing.

REFERENCES

Aristotle. (1947). Posterior Analytics (G. R. G. Mure, Trans.). In R. McKeon (Ed.), *Introduction to Aristotle* (pp. 9–109). New York: Random House.
Aristotle. (1984). Categories (J. L. Ackrill, Trans.). In J. Barnes (Ed.), *The complete works of Aristotle,* (pp. 3–24). Princeton, NJ: Princeton University Press.

Armstrong, S. L., Gleitman, L. R., & Gleitman, H. (1983). What some concepts might not be. *Cognition, 13,* 263–308.

Ayer, A. J. (Ed.). (1959). *Logical positivism.* Glencoe, Ill: Free Press.

Barsalou, L. W., & Medin, D. L. (1986). Concepts: Static definitions or context-dependent representations? *Cahiers de Psychologie Cognitive, 6,* 187–202.

Becker, C. H. (1983). A conceptualization of concept. *Nursing Papers, 15,* 51–58.

Boyd, C. (1985). Toward an understanding of mother-daughter identification using concept analysis. *Advances in Nursing Science, 7*(3), 78–86.

Carnap, R. (1956). *Meaning and necessity.* Chicago: University of Chicago Press.

Chinn, P. L., & Jacobs, M. K. (1987). *Theory and nursing: A systematic approach* (2nd ed.). St. Louis: Mosby.

Chinn, P. L., & Kramer, M. (1991). *Theory and nursing: A systematic approach* (3rd ed.). St. Louis: Mosby.

Descartes, R. (1960). Meditations on first philosophy. In M. C. Beardsley (Ed.), *The European philosophers from Descartes to Nietzsche* (pp. 25–96). New York: Random House. (Original work published 1644)

Diers, D. (1979). *Research in nursing practice.* Philadelphia: J. B. Lippincott.

Duffy, M. E. (1987). The concept of adaptation: Examining alternatives for the study of nursing phenomena. *Scholarly Inquiry for Nursing Practice, 1,* 179–192.

Duldt, B. W., & Giffin, K. (1985). *Theoretical perspectives for nursing.* Boston: Little, Brown.

Fehr, B. (1988). Prototype analysis of the concepts of love and commitment. *Journal of Personality and Social Psychology, 55,* 557–579.

Forsyth, G. L. (1980). Analysis of the concept of empathy: Illustration of one approach. *Advances in Nursing Science, 2*(2), 33–42.

Frege G. (1952a). Grundgesetze der Arithmetik (P. T. Geach, Trans.). In P. Geach & M. Black (Eds.), *Translations from the philosophical writings of Gottlob Frege* (pp. 159–181). Oxford: Basil Blackwell.

Frege, G. (1952b). On concept and object (P. T. Geach, Trans.). In P. Geach & M. Black (Eds.), *Translations from the philosophical writings of Gottlob Frege* (pp. 42–55). Oxford: Basil Blackwell.

Gibson, C. H. (1991). A concept analysis of empowerment. *Journal of Advanced Nursing, 16,* 354–361.

Hallett, G. (1967). *Wittgenstein's definition of meaning as use.* New York: Fordham University Press.

Hardy, M. K. (1974). Theories: Components, development, evaluation. *Nursing Research, 23,* 100–107.

Hartnack, J. (1965). *Wittgenstein and modern philosophy* (M. Cranston, Trans.). New York: New York University Press.

Jacox, A. (1974). Theory construction in nursing: An overview. *Nursing Research, 23,* 4–13.

Kant, I. (1965). *Critique of pure reason* (N. K. Smith, Trans.). New York: St. Martin's Press. (Original work published 1781)

Keck, J. F. (1986). Terminology of theory development. In A. Marriner (Ed.), *Nursing theorists and their work* (pp. 15–23). St. Louis: Mosby.

Kim, H. S. (1983). *The nature of theoretical thinking in nursing.* Norwalk, Conn: Appleton-Century-Crofts.

King, I. M. (1988). Concepts: Essential elements of theories. *Nursing Science Quarterly, 1,* 22–25.

Knafl, K. A., & Deatrick, J. A. (1986). How families manage chronic conditions: An analysis of the concept of normalization. *Research in Nursing & Health, 9,* 215–222.

Laudan, L. (1977). *Progress and its problems.* Berkeley: University of California Press.

Locke, J. (1975). *An essay concerning human understanding.* Oxford: Oxford University Press. (Original work published 1690)

Matteson, P., & Hawkins, J. W. (1990). Concept analysis of decision making. *Nursing Forum, 25*(2), 4–10.

McCloskey, M. E., & Glucksberg, S. (1978). Natural categories: Well defined or fuzzy sets? *Memory & Cognition, 6,* 462–472.

Medin, D. L. (1989). Concepts and conceptual structure. *American Psychologist, 44,* 1469–1481.

Medin, D. L., & Schaffer, M. M. (1978). Context theory of classification learning. *Psychological Review, 85,* 207–238.

Meize-Grochowski, R. (1984). An analysis of the concept of trust. *Journal of Advanced Nursing, 9,* 563–572.

Meleis, A. I. (1985). *Theoretical nursing.* Philadelphia: J. B. Lippincott.

Oden, G. C., & Lopes, L. (1982). On the internal structure of fuzzy subjective categories. In R. R. Yager (Ed.), *Recent developments in fuzzy set and possibility theory* (pp. 75–89). Elmsford, NY: Pergamon.

Rawnsley, M. M. (1980). The concept of privacy. *Advances in Nursing Science, 2*(2), 25–31.

Rew, L. (1986). Intuition: Concept analysis of a group phenomenon. *Advances in Nursing Science, 8*(2), 21–28.

Rodgers, B. L. (1989a). Concepts, analysis, and the development of nursing knowledge: The evolutionary cycle. *Journal of Advanced Nursing, 14,* 330–335.

Rodgers, B. L. (1989b). The use and application of concepts in nursing: The case of health policy (Doctoral dissertation, University of Virginia, 1987). *Dissertation Abstracts International, 49–11B,* 4756.

Rorty, R. (1979). *Philosophy and the mirror of nature.* Princeton, NJ: Princeton University.

Russell, B. (1914). *Our knowledge of the external world.* Chicago: Open Court.

Ryle, G. (1949). *The concept of mind.* Chicago: University of Chicago Press.

Ryle, G. (1971a). Systematically misleading expressions. In *Collected papers* (Vol. 2, pp. 39–62). London: Hutchinson.

Ryle, G. (1971b). The theory of meaning. In *Collected papers* (Vol. 2, pp. 350–372). London: Hutchinson.

Ryle, G. (1971c). Thinking thoughts and having concepts. In *Collected papers* (Vol. 2, pp. 446–450). London: Hutchinson.

Ryle, G. (1971d). Use, usage and meaning. In *Collected papers* (Vol. 2, pp. 407–414). London: Hutchinson.

Schlick, M. (1959). The turning point in philosophy (D. Rynin, Trans.). In A. J. Ayer (Ed.), *Logical positivism* (pp. 53–59). Glencoe, Ill: Free Press.

Silva, M. C., & Rothbart, D. R. (1983). An analysis of changing trends in philosophies of science on nursing theory development and testing. *Advances in Nursing Science, 6,* 1–13.

Simmons, S. J. (1989). Health: A concept analysis. *International Journal of Nursing Studies, 26,* 155–161.

Smith, E. E., & Medin, D. L. (1981). *Categories and concepts.* Cambridge, Mass: Harvard University Press.

Tadd, W., & Chadwick, R. (1989). Philosophical analysis and its value to the nurse teacher. *Nurse Education Today, 9,* 155–160.

Toulmin, S. (1972). *Human understanding.* Princeton, NJ: Princeton University Press.

Walker, L. O., & Avant, K. C. (1983). *Strategies for theory construction in nursing.* Norwalk, Conn: Appleton & Lange.

Walker, L. O., & Avant, K. C. (1988). *Strategies for theory construction in nursing* (2nd ed.). Norwalk, Conn: Appleton-Century-Crofts.

Watson, J. (1979). *Nursing: The philosophy and science of caring.* Boston: Little, Brown.

Webster, G., Jacox, A., & Baldwin, B. (1981). Nursing theory and the ghost of the received view. In J. C. McCloskey & H. K. Grace (Eds.), *Current issues in nursing* (pp. 26–35). Boston: Blackwell Scientific.

Westra, B. L., & Rodgers, B. L. (1991). The concept of integration: A foundation for evaluating outcomes of nursing care. *Journal of Professional Nursing, 7,* 277–282.

Wilson, J. (1963). *Thinking with concepts.* London: Cambridge University Press.

Wittgenstein, L. (1968). *Philosophical investigations* (3rd ed.; G. E. M. Anscombe, Trans.). New York: Macmillan. (Original work published 1953)

Wittgenstein, L. (1979). *Notebooks: 1914–1916* (2nd ed.; G. E. M. Anscombe, Trans.). Chicago: University of Chicago Press.

Wittgenstein, L. (1981). *Tractatus logico-philosophicus* (D. F. Pears & B. F. McGuinness, Trans.). London: Routledge & Kegan Paul. (Original work published 1921)

Chapter 3

Knowledge Synthesis and Concept Development in Nursing

KATHLEEN A. KNAFL AND JANET A. DEATRICK

*I*n a recent editorial in *Nursing Research,* Florence Downs (1989) criticized the noncumulative nature of nursing research stating, "We all need to become much more sensitive to the fact that 'stop and go' activity ends in proliferation of isolated findings. Classification and synthesis remain essential to furthering realistic theory development and an understanding of how conditions are related within a nursing context" (p. 323). While not disputing the validity of Downs' critique, it also is true that there has been a growing interest in knowledge synthesis in nursing. Nurse scholars have both utilized and developed a variety of approaches to knowledge synthesis. To date, much of the work in this area has been directed to concept analysis.

Nursing has evidenced a long-standing recognition of the importance of concept development for the advancement of nursing theory and practice (Hardy, 1974; Jacox, 1974; Norris, 1982). Concept analysis was given a major impetus in the early 1980s when both Chinn and Jacobs (1983) and Walker and Avant (1983) published books on nursing theory that offered guidelines for conducting concept analysis. Since then, authors have continued to publish both guidelines for concept analysis and results of analyses (Chinn & Jacobs, 1987; Knafl & Deatrick, 1986, 1990; Rew, 1986; Rodgers, 1989a, 1989b; Schwartz-Barcott & Kim, 1986; Tilden, 1985; Walker & Avant, 1988). Concept analysis typically entails synthesizing existing views of a concept and distinguishing it from other concepts. There are also other approaches to knowledge synthesis including a variety of approaches for reviewing the literature (Artinian, 1982; Cooper, 1982, 1984, 1989; Ganong, 1987; Noblit & Hare, 1988).

Little attention has been given to comparing the relative merits of these different approaches to knowledge synthesis. As a result, readers may not understand why a particular approach was selected, and authors may not consider the full range of approaches when undertaking a knowledge synthesis project. The aim of this chapter is to present an overview of several broad approaches to knowledge synthesis and a more detailed comparison of approaches to concept analysis and development.

Approaches to Knowledge Synthesis

The strategies summarized in Table 3–1 are directed toward evaluating knowledge development in a particular domain. Using each, the analyst critically reviews literature, occasionally gathers data, and draws conclusions regarding what is known and what further work needs to be done in a particular area of interest. If successful, the synthesis conveys to the reader the "state of the art" in a given area.

LITERATURE REVIEWS

Guidelines for conducting integrative reviews and critiques of existing reviews can be found in the literature. Both Jackson (1980) and Cooper (1982, 1984, 1989) distinguished various types of integrative reviews and conceptualized integrative reviews as a research process. Jackson (1980) maintained that such reviews could serve a variety of substantive, methodological, and theoretical purposes. Similarly, Cooper (1989) noted that "reviews can focus on research outcomes, research methods, theories, and/or applications" (p. 13). Ganong (1987) provided guidelines for conducting integrative reviews and critiqued 17 published reviews of nursing research. He emphasized the importance of being explicit in the review as to one's purpose, sampling design, and data collection methods.

Other authors (Abraham & Schultz, 1983; Devine & Cook, 1983; Glass, 1976; Smith & Naftel, 1984) addressed how statistical techniques can be used in integrative literature reviews. Glass (1976) described this approach, known as *meta-analysis:*

> *Meta-analysis refers to the analysis of analyses. I use it to refer to the statistical analysis of a large collection of analysis results from individual studies for the purpose of integrating the findings. (p. 3)*

These publications cite the results of specific meta-analyses: Brown, 1988; Devine & Cook, 1983; Johnson, 1988; Schwartz, Moody, Yarandi, & Anderson, 1987. Smith and Naftel (1984) listed existing analyses. In the past several years, the emphasis has shifted in meta-analysis from the single purpose of measuring effect size to a more encompassing goal of concept clarification (Booth-Kewley & Friedman, 1987).

Noblit and Hare (1988) recently outlined a framework for synthesizing the results of qualitative studies, a technique they termed *meta-ethnography.* Meta-ethnography is an inductive approach that Noblit and Hare describe as a series of overlapping phases relying on the technique of meta-

Table 3-1 *Strategies for Synthesizing Knowledge*

STRATEGY	PURPOSE	DATA SOURCE	PROPONENTS
Literature Review Integrative Meta-Analysis Meta-Ethnography Conceptual Mapping	Knowledge synthesis/ aggregation	Literature	Artinian (1982); Cooper (1982, 1984, 1989); Devine & Cook (1983); Ganong (1987); Glass (1976); Jackson, (1980); Noblit & Hare (1988)
Concept Analysis	Identification, clarification, or refinement of a concept	Literature; empirical data; constructed cases	Chinn & Jacobs (Kramer), (1983, 1987, 1991); Rodgers (1989a); Sartori (1984); Schwartz-Barcott & Kim (1986); Walker & Avant (1983, 1988); Wilson (1969).

phoric reduction to translate the interpretations of one qualitative study into the interpretations of another. As in meta-analysis, the reviewer synthesizes the results of existing research. However, meta-ethnography is viewed by its developers as unique from other approaches to knowledge synthesis. Noblit and Hare (1988) maintained.

We use the term meta-ethnography to highlight our proposal as an interpretive alternative to research synthesis. For us, the meta *in metaethnography means something different than it does in meta-analysis. It refers not to developing overarching generalizations but, rather, translations of qualitative studies into one another. (p. 25)*

Noblit and Hare highlight their description with examples throughout the text. Certainly, meta-ethnography offers a promising approach for integrating the results of the numerous ethnographic, grounded theory, and phenomenological studies published in nursing.

In an effort to understand the comparative merits of quantitative and qualitative approaches to conducting integrative reviews, Brown and Hellings (1988) compared the results of their meta-analysis of studies of maternal-infant attachment to Lamb and Hwang's (1982) qualitative review of the same topic. They found that important advantages of meta-analysis are avoidance of type II errors and investigator bias. On the other hand, qualitative reviews give the reader a better sense of individual studies, combine results from methodologically diverse studies, allow for the investigation of the influence of multiple variables, and are not limited by the author's failure to report certain statistics. Given the distinct advantages of the approaches, Brown and Hellings (1988) concluded that both types of reviews are useful.

In contrast to the analytical techniques associated with integrative reviews and the specific statistical techniques of meta-analysis, Artinian (1982) developed conceptual mapping for depicting "the relationships among variables linking the independent variables to the dependent variable" (p. 379). As described by Artinian, the purpose of conceptual mapping is to clarify the research problem in the context of proposal development. Conceptual mapping requires the explicit identification of concepts of interest and facilitates identification of how these concepts have been related to one another in previous research. Artinian described conceptual mapping as an especially useful educational technique for graduate students embarking on their first research project, and provided detailed examples of conceptual maps completed by former students. Unlike other synthesizing approaches, conceptual mapping was not presented as resulting in a "stand alone" scholarly outcome.

Although the aforementioned techniques offer general and specialized approaches for knowledge synthesis, they do not explicitly address concept clarification and development as a primary goal. Methods for concept analysis fill that gap.

Approaches to Concept Analysis

As shown in Table 3–2, scholars have developed several approaches to concept analysis. While all approaches share a common focus on concept clarification, authors linked their approaches to distinct intellectual underpinnings and identified somewhat different analytic goals. Moreover, they specified varying steps or phases as comprising the work of concept analysis. Table 3–2 summarizes these differences across the approaches with regard to the following: intellectual underpinnings, analytic purposes, and analytic steps or phases. Exemplar references for each approach are also included in the table.

CHINN AND JACOBS

Chinn and Jacobs (1983, 1987) described their approach to concept analysis as an adaptation of Wilson's (1969) method. Like Wilson's, their approach relies heavily on the development of exemplary cases (model, contrary, related, borderline) that are used to identify the defining criteria of the concept. Criteria, which were described as always tentative, reflect what is learned about the concept from developing cases and from selectively reviewing the literature.

Forsyth (1980) used this approach in analyzing the concept of empathy. She presented a model case of empathy followed by a discussion of defining criteria for the concept as reflected in the model case. Her discussion incorporated validating evidence from the literature. The concept and the provisional criteria were further refined and expanded through the presentation and analysis of contrary, related, and borderline cases and through further review of the literature. Forsyth described her review of the literature as selective and not exhaustive.

Throughout her presentation, Forsyth (1980) emphasized the simultaneous nature of the activities of concept analysis and stated, "The techniques are not necessarily used in step-by-step fashion; rather they tend to emerge simultaneously once the initial steps of analysis have been undertaken" (p. 34). She noted that concept analysis is best done as a collaborative endeavor.

In the 1991 edition of *Theory and Nursing: A Systematic Approach,* Chinn and Jacobs (now Kramer) introduced several refinements to their approach to concept analysis, which is presented as a strategy for creating meaning. They stated that "conceptual meaning is something that is created. It does not 'exist' as an 'out there' reality, but it is deliberately formed from empiric experience" (p. 80).

Table 3-2 *Approaches to Concept Analysis/Development*

APPROACH	UNDERPINNINGS	PURPOSE	PHASES/STEPS	EXAMPLE
Chinn & Jacobs (1983, 1987)	Wilson (1969)	"To arrive at a tentative definition of the concept and a set of tentative criteria by which one can judge whether or not the empirical phenomena associated with the concept exist in a particular situation" (Chinn & Jacobs, 1983, p. 90).	1. Identify concept 2. Specify aims 3. Examine definitions 4. Construct cases 5. Test cases 6. Formulate criteria	Forsyth (1980)/ Empathy
Chinn & Kramer (1991)	Wilson (1969); Walker & Avant (1988)	"Produce a tentative definition of the concept and a set of tentative criteria for determining if the concept 'exists' in a particular situation" (Chinn & Kramer, 1991, p. 88).	1. Select a concept 2. Clarify purpose 3. Identify data sources 4. Explore context and values 5. Formulate criteria	None
Walker & Avant (1983, 1988)	Wilson (1969)	"To distinguish between the defining attributes of a concept and its irrelevant attributes" (Walker & Avant, 1988, p. 35).	1. Select concept 2. Determine aim of analysis 3. Identify all uses of concept 4. Determine defining attributes	Boyd (1985)/ Mother-daughter identification; Rew (1986)/Intuition

| | | 5. Construct a model case
6. Construct additional cases
7. Identify antecedents and consequences
8. Define empirical referents | |
| Rodgers (1989a) | To clarify the current use of a concept with attention to contextual and temporal aspects; to provide a clear conceptual foundation as a heuristic for further inquiry (Rodgers, 1989a; see chapter 6) | 1. Identify the concept of interest
2. Identify surrogate terms
3. Identify sample for data collection
4. Identify attributes of the concept
5. Identify references, antecedents, and consequences of concept
6. Identify related concepts
7. Identify a model case
8. Conduct interdisciplinary and temporal comparisons. | Price (1953); Rorty (1979); Toulmin (1972); Wittgenstein (1968) | Rodgers (1989a, 1989b)/Health Policy; Cowles & Rodgers (see chapter 7)/ Grief; Westra & Rodgers (1991) Integration |

Table continued on following page

Table 3–2 *Approaches to Concept Analysis/Development* Continued

APPROACH	UNDERPINNINGS	PURPOSE	PHASES/STEPS	EXAMPLE
Sartori (1984)	Ogden & Richards (1946)	"To arrive at a definition of the concept that is both adequate and harmonious" (Sartori, 1984, p. 56).	1. Reconstruct concept 2. Select designating term 3. Reconceptualize the concept	Sartori (1984)/consensus, development, ethnicity, integration, political culture, power, revolution
Schwartz-Barcott & Kim (1986)	Reynolds (1971); Schatzman & Strauss (1973); Wilson (1969)	"To identify, analyze, and refine concepts in the initial stage of theory development" (Schwartz-Barcott & Kim, 1986, p. 91).	1. Theoretical phase 2. Fieldwork phase 3. Analytical phase	Madden (1990)/therapeutic alliance; Carboni (1990)/homelessness

As shown in Table 3–2, Chinn and Kramer credited both Wilson (1969) and Walker and Avant (1983, 1988) as influencing their approach to what they termed *concept clarification.* While the underlying purpose and steps of the clarification process remained similar to the first two editions, the authors expanded the data sources they recommended considering as part of the analysis. Under data sources they discussed definitions, cases (model, contrary, related, and borderline), visual images, popular and classical literature, music, professional literature, and people. The presentation of data sources was couched in an explicit recognition of empirics, ethics, aesthetics, and personal knowing as distinct ways of knowing. In their discussion of the use of multiple data sources, Chinn and Kramer argue that "although case techniques that are associated with creating conceptual meaning are very useful, when they are supplemented with other data sources, a richer meaning for concepts evolves" (p. 93). Also new in this edition was their consideration of how the meaning of a concept varies across contexts and their recommendation that clarification strategies be adapted to the specific purpose of the analysis. Given the recency of the third edition, no examples of analyses using the refined approach are available.

WALKER AND AVANT

Walker and Avant (1983, 1988) identified concept analysis as one of three approaches to concept development. Other strategies included concept synthesis for the development of new concepts and concept derivation for the translation of concepts across disciplines.

Like Chinn and Jacobs (1983, 1987) and Chinn and Kramer (1991), this approach to concept analysis builds on Wilson's (1969) seminal work. As noted in Table 3–2, the approaches differ somewhat in the steps and ordering of the analytic process. Although the authors of these approaches pointed out that concept analysis usually does not proceed in a strictly linear fashion, their differential ordering of steps leads to a somewhat different emphasis in the analytic process. For Walker and Avant (1988), case construction followed identification of defining criteria and served to illustrate the presence or absence of the criteria across the concept of interest and related concepts; for Chinn and Jacobs (1987), case construction preceded formulation of defining criteria and played a key role in the defining process. Chinn and Kramer (1991) incorporated case construction as one of many possible data sources that contributed to the formulation of defining criteria. Walker and Avant included the specification of antecedents, consequences, and empirical referents as components of the analysis, while Chinn and Kramer encouraged the exploration of various contexts and values associated with the concept.

Boyd (1985) and Rew (1986) used Walker and Avant's approach to concept analysis to analyze mother-daughter identification (Boyd, 1985) and intuition (Rew, 1986). Both analyses followed the steps outlined by Walker and Avant. Rew did not explicitly state the aims of her analysis, but convincingly argued for the relevance of the concept of intuition for nursing practice and education. Boyd framed her analysis, as suggested by Walker and Avant (1983, 1988), in terms of its clinical origins and explicitly stated her overall purpose. Both authors' analyses included a review of selected literature. Defining attributes, antecedents, and consequences evolved from the literature review (Boyd, 1985; Rew, 1986) and from clinical experience (Boyd, 1985). Both authors constructed model and alternate cases to clarify and illustrate the defining attributes of the concepts they analyzed. The authors then identified empirical referents to "demonstrate the existence of the concept" (Boyd, 1985, p. 84). Finally, each author presented implications that were consistent with the aims of the analysis. Rew (1986) directed her discussion to practical issues related to nursing education and professional organizations, while Boyd (1985) discussed the implications for nursing practice, theory development, and research.

RODGERS

Rodgers (1989a) offered an approach to concept analysis that "overcomes difficulties with a positivistic or reductionistic view and that addresses contemporary concerns valuing dynamism and interrelationships within reality" (p. 332). Rodgers integrated the views of several prominent philosophers (Price, 1953; Rorty, 1979; Toulmin, 1972; Wittgenstein, 1953/1968) in developing her evolutionary view of concepts as continually subject to change, and as developing through significance, use, and application. *Significance* is "the concept's ability to assist in the resolution of problems, its ability to characterize phenomena adequately, thus furthering efforts toward the achievement of intellectual ideals" (Rodgers, 1989a, p. 332). Use of the concept refers to the manner in which it is employed and its application refers to actual instances of use. According to Rodgers, it is through the process of application that concepts are further refined and developed.

Rodgers maintained that her approach differs from traditional approaches to concept analysis in several important ways. She emphasized that the analytic process was nonlinear and involved a series of overlapping phases rather than sequential steps. Rodgers also maintained that the singular, fundamental purpose of concept analysis was to clarify the concept of interest. At the same time, she pointed out that such clarification was an essential dimension of nursing diagnosis development and clinical problem solving (see chapters 6 and 7). Moreover, she stated that only a model case should be presented, since the use of other types of cases such as contrary and borderline reflected a view of concepts as unchanging. She stated, "Such cases are not consistent with the view of concepts that underlies this revised method. Instead, their functions are addressed in the form of related concepts, a change that recognizes the interconnectedness of the world and the likelihood of change" (p. 333). Rodgers also favored identifying real-life model cases rather than constructing such cases solely for the purpose of the analysis. She contended, "A model case of a concept enhances the degree of clarification offered as a result of analysis by providing an everyday example that includes the attributes of the concept" (p. 334).

In a separate publication of the results of an analysis of the concept of health policy, Rodgers (1989b) employed her approach in order to clarify the current use of the concept. The analysis proceeded through a series of flexible phases rather than invariate steps and included a detailed account of procedures for sampling the literature. Based on her evolutionary view of concepts, she presented only an empirically based model case of the concept.

SARTORI

Sartori's approach to concept analysis builds on Ogden and Richards's (1946) work and focuses on words, meanings, and referents and the relationships among the three. Sartori's (1984) book, *Social Science Concepts: A Systematic Analysis,* included a description of his method of concept analysis as well as concept analyses by different authors on a variety of topics such as consensus, development, ethnicity, and power. Sartori described a three-step process in which the concept was reconstructed, named, and reconceptualized. Concept reconstruction entailed reviewing and synthesizing existing knowledge about the concept. Concept formation and reconceptualization encompassed selecting a term to name the concept, and then refining the concept. Sartori's approach does not use case presentations.

Although basing their analyses on Sartori's framework, authors who contributed concept analyses to his book employed somewhat different applications of his three-step process, adapting it to their purposes and to the body of literature related to the concept. In general, each author's analysis was based on a selective review of research literature. In their applications of Sartori's approach, authors typically used descriptive grids to summarize characteristics of the concept reflected in the literature. Figures were used to show the relationship between the concept of interest and related concepts.

For example, Jackson (1984) used Sartori's framework to analyze the concept of ethnicity. His analysis focused on existing definitions of the concept and the identification of empirical referents. Jackson (1984) noted that he selected definitions because they were "prominent in the literature on ethnicity and rather typical" (p. 219). As a result of this reconstruction phase of the analysis, he identified "core characteristics" of the concept. Based on these core characteristics, he named the concept "ethnic collectivities" and concluded his presentation with a series of summary definitions of the concept and related concepts such as ethnic category and ethnic group. Taken as a whole, Sartori's book provides a detailed elaboration of one approach to concept analysis and a series of diverse analyses exemplifying the wide-ranging applicability of the approach.

SCHWARTZ-BARCOTT AND KIM

Schwartz-Barcott and Kim (1986) presented a "hybrid model" for concept development that explicitly incorporated both theoretical and empirical activities. The hybrid approach consists of three sequential phases: theoretical, fieldwork, and final analytical. It builds on Reynolds's (1971) composite approach to the development of scientific knowledge, Wilson's (1969) approach to concept analysis, and Schatzman and Strauss's (1973) book *Field Research: Strategies for a Natural Sociology.*

During the theoretical phase, the literature is reviewed with an eye to selecting a working definition of the concept of interest. This working definition then serves to focus the fieldwork phase of concept development, which is "aimed at refining a concept that has been analyzed in the theoretical phase" (Schwartz-Barcott & Kim, 1986, p. 96). Refinement serves to validate and elaborate the concept through qualitative research. During the final analytical phase, the results from the two previous phases are integrated in order to define the concept and identify measurement issues and strategies. At this point, the concept's applicability and importance to nursing is evaluated.

The authors provided a detailed example of how the hybrid model was used by a graduate student to develop the concept of withdrawal. To date, the hybrid model has been used primarily as an educational device for students working on their master's research projects and doctoral dissertations (D. Schwartz-Barcott, personal communication, March 3, 1989). Recently Madden (1990) used the hybrid model to analyze and develop further the concept of therapeutic alliance. Based on a review of the literature, Madden formulated a working definition of the concept that she subsequently used to direct her observations of interactions between community health nurses and their clients. Observational data were analyzed systematically and used to expand the initial working definition of the concept. During the final analysis phase, the revised definition of therapeutic alliance was discussed in terms of existing nursing theories. Although preceding the hybrid model, Avant's (1979) discussion of maternal attachment provides another example of combining theoretical and empirical data to identify and refine defining criteria for a concept.

DISCUSSION

Scholars engaged in knowledge synthesis have a wide range of approaches at their disposal. These approaches address a variety of purposes. While some are geared to knowledge aggregation in a substantive area, others focus on refining and clarifying a single concept. Some, such as conceptual mapping and hybrid concept development, have been initiated and applied primarily as educational techniques for beginning researchers in graduate programs. Other approaches, such as integrative reviews and concept analysis, have a long history of mainstream scientific endeavors. Two of the techniques, meta-analysis and meta-ethnography, are relatively new. Given the variety of approaches, it is best to look at the strategies presented in Tables 3–1 and 3–2 as a menu of possibilities that should be fit to one's purposes and desired outcome at the outset. The rationale for using a particular strategy should be justified as it will help to clarify the approach and the nature of the phenomenon being explored in the synthesis activity.

While current information is available on each approach, the extent to which they have been applied by nurse scholars varies considerably. There are numerous published examples in nursing of integrative reviews, meta-analyses and concept analyses. In contrast, few authors have reported meta-ethnographies, hybrid-model concept development, or conceptual mapping. It is hoped that an awareness of such alternative strategies will result in their use and further development.

Regarding concept analysis, explicit comparison of the approaches revealed important differences among them. As different methods of concept analysis were explored, it became apparent that the nature of the literature review and the use of illustrative cases varied considerably.

Chinn and Jacobs (1983, 1987) said little about the literature review stage of the analysis, and the applications of their approach by others tended to rely heavily on the presentation of cases. Typically, the cases were constructed early in the analysis to help identify defining criteria, which were tested and refined throughout the course of analysis. Chinn and Jacobs recommended the development of multiple types of cases (e.g., model, contrary, related) and did not distinguish between empirically based cases and those created for the purpose of the analysis.

Chinn and Kramer (1991) identified cases (model, contrary, related, and borderline) as one of several data sources to be used in generating and refining defining criteria. Like the other sources of data, cases were used to stimulate thinking about the concept. While they emphasized using many diverse sources of data, Chinn and Kramer (1991) gave few guidelines for reviewing or synthesizing such data. They maintained that concept clarification should be a thoughtful, systematic process.

Walker and Avant (1983, 1988) stressed the centrality of the literature review to concept analysis. Although they did not provide explicit guidelines for carrying out such a review, they encouraged the analyst to do extensive reading in widely varying sources and to maintain a systematic record of the various ways in which the concept was used in the literature. They maintained that cases usually were used to illustrate the defining criteria of a concept. They acknowledged, however, that with a new concept, cases may be used to help identify defining criteria. Like Chinn and Jacobs, they recommended the development of multiple types of cases.

Rodgers (1989a) also emphasized the importance of the literature review. Moreover, unlike other authors, she specified guidelines for sampling the literature and suggested that a model case be identified at the end of the analysis to clarify and illustrate the concept. She advised that the model case be based on an everyday example of the concept, a position she maintained was consistent with her evolutionary view of concepts. Cases are not used to identify defining attributes in this approach.

The literature review was also a major aspect of Sartori's approach and comprised the initial phase of the analysis, concept reconstruction. While he did not specify guidelines for sampling the literature, he did suggest that the analyst note differences in usage across disciplinary boundaries. He did not discuss the use of case development in his approach.

Like Sartori, Schwartz-Barcott and Kim recommended initiating their hybrid approach to concept analysis with a review of the literature. Although, they did not address the topic of case development, their empirical phase entailed data collection for the purpose of both developing the concept and illustrating its *real world* existence. Their approach speaks to the importance of balancing reliance on existing literature and new data when the intent is the further refinement of a relatively new or undeveloped concept.

The strategies described in this paper provide an overview of selected approaches to knowledge synthesis and concept development. They accommodate a wide variety of purposes and knowledge bases. Most can be used either to prepare for further research or as free-standing scholarly endeavors. We recommend that the strategies described be viewed as a "menu of possibilities." Selection of a specific item from the menu might reasonably begin by considering the scope of your interests. If the focus of interest is a particular concept rather than a broader substantive or theoretical area, you can consider menu items specific to concept analysis. Within this narrower range of choices, it is important to keep in mind that different approaches to concept analysis are geared to somewhat different purposes. Rodgers (1989a, 1989b) and Sartori (1984) focus their attention solely on concept clarification; Chinn and Jacobs (1983, 1987), Chinn and Kramer (1991), and Walker and Avant (1983, 1988) cite a wider range of purposes including such things as developing an operational definition or refining a nursing diagnosis. Chinn and Kramer (1991) point out that concept analysis is a way to create conceptual meaning and that different purposes can advance that more general goal. Schwartz-Barcott and Kim's (1986) approach is specifically geared to using formal concept analysis as a starting point for further empirical work geared to elaborating the concept.

Persons interested in synthesizing knowledge in a more encompassing substantive or theoretical domain can choose from a variety of approaches for conducting reviews of the literature. If the field of interest is characterized primarily by experimental studies, meta-analysis may be an ideal way to synthesize knowledge. In contrast, meta-ethnography is especially tailored to fields of study dominated by qualitative work. The conventional integrative review provides a useful alternative for scholars who do not choose to limit their review to studies using a particular type of methodology. Whatever approach to knowledge synthesis is finally chosen, scholars embarking on such a project are encouraged to consider the full array of possibilities and to select the one most suited to their purposes.

REFERENCES

Abraham, I. L., & Schultz, S. (1983). Univariate statistical models for meta-analysis. *Nursing Research, 32,* 312–315.

Artinian, B. (1982). Conceptual mapping: Development of the strategy. *Western Journal of Nursing Research, 4,* 379–393.

Avant, K. (1979). Nursing diagnosis: Maternal attachment. *Advances in Nursing Science, 2*(1), 45–55.

Booth-Kewley, S., & Friedman, H. S. (1987). Psychological predictors of heart disease: A quantitative review. *Psychological Bulletin, 101,* 343–362.

Boyd, C. (1985). Toward an understanding of mother-daughter identification using concept analysis. *Advances in Nursing Science, 7*(3), 78–86.

Brown, S. A. (1988). Effect of educational interventions on diabetes care: A meta-analysis of findings. *Nursing Research, 37,* 223–230.

Brown, M., & Hellings, P. (1988). A case study of qualitative versus quantitative reviews: The maternal-infant bonding controversy. *Journal of Pediatric Nursing, 4,* 104–111.

Carboni, J. (1990). Homelessness among the institutionalized elderly. *Journal of Gerontological Nursing, 16,* 32–37.

Chinn, P., & Jacobs, M. (1983). *Theory and nursing: A systematic approach.* St. Louis: Mosby.

Chinn, P., & Jacobs, M. (1987). *Theory and nursing: A systematic approach* (2nd ed.). St. Louis: Mosby.

Chinn, P., & Kramer, M. (1991). *Theory and nursing: A systematic approach* (3rd ed.). St. Louis: Mosby.

Cooper, H. M. (1982). Scientific guidelines for conducting integrative research reviews. *Review of Educational Research, 52,* 291–302.

Cooper, H. M. (1984). *The integrative research review: A systematic approach.* Beverly Hills: Sage.

Cooper, H. (1989). *Integrating research: A guide for literature reviews* (2nd ed.). Beverly Hills: Sage.

Devine, E. C., & Cook, T. D. (1983). A meta-analytic analysis of psychoeducational interventions on length of postsurgical hospital stay. *Nursing Research, 32,* 267–274.

Downs, F. (1989). New questions and new answers. *Nursing Research, 38,* 323.

Forsyth, G. L. (1980). Analysis of the concept of empathy: Illustration of one approach. *Advances in Nursing Science, 2*(2), 33–42.

Ganong, L. H. (1987). Integrative reviews of nursing research. *Research in Nursing and Health, 10,* 1–11.

Glass, G. (1976). Primary, secondary, and meta analysis of research. *Educational Researcher, 5,* 3–8.

Hardy, M. K. (1974). Theories: Components, development, evaluation. *Nursing Research, 23,* 100–107.

Jackson, G. B. (1980). Methods for integrative reviews. *Reviews of Educational Research, 50,* 438–460.

Jackson, R. (1984). Ethnicity. In G. Sartori (Ed.), *Social science concepts: A systematic approach* (pp. 205–233). Beverly Hills: Sage.

Jacox, A. (1974). Theory construction in nursing: An overview. *Nursing Research, 23,* 4–13.

Johnson, J. H. (1988). Differences in the performances of baccalaureate, associate degree, and diploma nurses: A meta-analysis. *Research in Nursing and Health, 11,* 183–198.

Knafl, K. A., & Deatrick, J. A. (1986). How families manage chronic conditions: An analysis of the concept of normalization. *Research in Nursing and Health, 9,* 215–222.

Knafl, K. A., & Deatrick, J. A. (1990). Family management style: Concept analysis and development. *Journal of Pediatric Nursing, 5,* 4–14.

Lamb, M., & Hwang, C. (1982). Maternal attachment and mother-neonate bonding: A critical review. In M. Lamb & A. Brown (Eds.), *Advances in developmental psychology* (Vol. 2: pp. 1–39). Hillsdale, NJ: Erlbaum.

Madden, B. (1990). The hybrid model for concept development: Its value for the study of therapeutic alliance. *Advances in Nursing Science, 12*(3), 75–87.

Noblit, G., & Hare, R. (1988). *Meta-ethnography: Synthesizing qualitative studies.* Beverly Hills: Sage.

Norris, C. M. (Eds.). (1982). *Concept clarification in nursing.* Germantown, Md: Aspen Systems.

Ogden, C. K., & Richards, I. A. (1946). *The meaning of meaning.* New York: Harcourt Brace Jovanovich.

Price, H. H. (1953). *Thinking and experience.* London: Hutchinson House.

Rew, L. (1986). Intuition: Concept analysis of a group phenomenon. *Advances in Nursing Science, 8*(2), 21–28.

Reynolds, P. (1971). *A primer in theory construction.* Indianapolis: Bobbs-Merrill.

Rodgers, B. L. (1989a). Concepts, analysis, and the development of nursing knowledge: The evolutionary cycle. *Journal of Advanced Nursing, 14,* 330–335.

Rodgers, B. L. (1989b). Exploring health policy as a concept. *Western Journal of Nursing Research, 11,* 694–702.

Rorty, R. (1979). *Philosophy and the mirror of nature.* Princeton, NJ: Princeton University.

Sartori, G. (1984). *Social science concepts: A systematic analysis.* Beverly Hills: Sage.

Schatzman, L., & Strauss, A. (1973). *Field research: Strategies for a natural sociology.* Englewood Cliffs, NJ: Prentice Hall.

Schwartz, R., Moody, L., Yarandi, H., & Anderson, G. (1987). A Meta-analysis of critical outcome variables in non-nutritive sucking in preterm infants. *Nursing Research, 36,* 292–297.

Schwartz-Barcott, D., & Kim, H. (1986). A hybrid model for concept development. In P. L. Chinn (Ed.), *Nursing research methodology: Issues and implementation* (pp. 91–101). Rockville, Md: Aspen.

Smith, C., & Naftel, D. (1984). Meta-analysis: A perspective for research synthesis. *Image, 16,* 9–13.

Tilden, V. (1985). Issues of conceptualization and measurement of social support in the construction of nursing theory. *Research in Nursing and Health, 8,* 199–206.

Toulmin, S. (1972). *Human understanding.* Princeton, NJ: Princeton University Press.

Walker, L. O., & Avant, K. C. (1983). *Strategies for theory construction in nursing.* Norwalk, Conn: Appleton-Century-Crofts.

Walker, L. O., & Avant, K. (1988). *Strategies for theory construction in nursing* (2nd ed.). Norwalk, Conn: Appleton and Lange.

Westra, B. L., & Rodgers, B. L. (1991). The concept of integration: A foundation for evaluating outcomes of nursing care. *Journal of Professional Nursing, 7,* 277–282.

Wilson, J. (1969). *Thinking with concepts.* New York: Cambridge University Press.

Wittgenstein, L. (1968). *Philosophical investigations* (3rd ed.). (G. E. M. Anscombe, Trans.). New York: MacMillan. (Original work published 1953)

Chapter 4

The Wilson Method of
Concept Analysis

KAY C. AVANT

*I*n the preface to his book *Thinking with Concepts* (1963), Wilson explained that the text was written expressly to be "worked through" by students (in particular, his sixth form—or high school—students) in an effort to gain skill in answering questions of a conceptual nature. He proposed that analysis of concepts "gives framework and purposiveness to thinking that might otherwise meander indefinitely and purposelessly among the vast marshes of intellect and culture" (p. ix). Throughout the book, Wilson continued to emphasize that concept analysis is a technique that aids the user in clear thinking and communication.

Wilson spent the first part of his book discussing the methods and techniques of concept analysis. Parts 2 and 4 are extensive examples of the use of the techniques and some practice exercises for the reader or student. Part 3 is a brief discussion of the links between philosophy and concept analysis. For further explanations of Parts 2, 3, and 4, the reader is referred to the original source. For the purposes of this chapter, Part 1 of Wilson's book will be the primary source of information.

In this chapter, the techniques Wilson advocated will be explained and then will be used in examining a concept of interest to nursing. The concept to be examined will be *science.*

Wilson listed eleven steps in concept analysis:

1. Isolating questions of concept
2. Finding right answers
3. Model cases
4. Contrary cases
5. Related cases
6. Borderline cases
7. Invented cases
8. Social context
9. Underlying anxiety
10. Practical results
11. Results in language

Each of these eleven steps will be considered separately in the following pages and the nursing example used to illustrate each.

Isolating Questions of Concept

Wilson distinguished among three types of questions: questions of fact, questions of values, and questions of concept. Questions of fact can be answered with knowledge that is already available in some form. Questions of value are answered based on moral principles present within an individual or a society. Questions of concept, however, are about meaning; the way questions of concept are answered depends entirely on the angle from which the analyst is looking at them. Wilson uses the example of the question "Is a whale a fish?" (1963, p. 4). The answer to this question, according to Wilson, might vary depending on whether the one posing the question was a marine biologist or working in the ministry of agriculture and fisheries. To the marine biologist, since a whale is a mammal, it may not "count" as a fish. On the other hand, to someone from the ministry of agriculture and fisheries, a whale probably would be considered a fish since it swims in the sea with the other fish.

Wilson (1963) made it clear that questions are rarely in their pure form. Many questions are mixed; that is, they require more than one type of analysis in order to answer them. He gave the example of the question "Should people in mental asylums [*sic*] ever be punished?" (p. 23). To answer this question clearly, the analyst must know some facts about the kinds of people usually found in psychiatric hospitals, know what is meant by the concept of punishment, and make a value or moral judgement about whether punishment is appropriate for such people. Therefore, before embarking on a concept analysis, the analyst should be sure that the question being answered is one of concept and not one of fact or value.

What is of concern in questions of concept are the actual and possible uses of words. When asking a question of concept, one is asking "what counts" as the concept or "what criteria" are being used to determine the meaning of the concept. Wilson suggests that one should take concepts seriously by becoming self-conscious about how words are used.

Concepts, and the words used to express them, are meant to serve human purposes and to do so efficiently. The way a person decides to use a word is of considerable importance. Words often do not have a single meaning. Individuals in various geographical regions may use the same word, but the meaning may be entirely different. Meanings for words change over time and over generations. For instance, in the West and Southwest, a *dude* meant someone who was unfamiliar with a working farm or ranch and who often wore inappropriate clothing for such work. A *dude* was an object of derision. Now, a *dude* is "cool" to youngsters, thanks to a popular movie concerning mutant turtles and Bart Simpson.

Two disciplines may use the same label for a concept that may have different meanings in those two disciplines. For instance, the concept of *support* is somewhat different in architecture and in nursing. In architecture, the concept of support is used to express the idea of a physical structure underlying and upholding an edifice. In nursing, however, the concept of support is more often used to mean emotional or social assistance.

A question often asked in nursing is "Is nursing a science or an art?" A corollary to this question is "Should nursing be a science?" These two questions demonstrate Wilson's ideas about questions of fact, values, and concept. The first question is a question of concept. The second one is a question of value. The issue of whether nursing *should* be a science is not one that can be answered by either facts or by analysis of the concept. It can only be answered by examining values. However, the question about whether nursing is an art or a science *is* a question of concept. It requires an understanding of what nursing is and also what science is. What counts as nursing? What counts as science? These questions can be answered by determining what nursing is and what science is and then comparing the essential elements of nursing to the essential elements of science to determine the fit. For the purposes of this chapter, we will assume that the reader already knows the essential elements of nursing and thus will focus only on the concept of science.

"Right" Answers

Often questions about concepts do not have a single "right" answer. It may be inappropriate to speak of *the* meaning of a word. It is also unwise, however, to assume that concepts are completely limitless and may be defined any way one pleases. Some ways in which a concept is used are closer to the heart or core of the concept than others. The uses that are somehow farther from the core are frequently metaphors, extensions, derivations, or borderline uses of the concept. The analyst needs to determine which elements are essential to the core of the concept and which are not.

A concept may be used in two contexts, each of which implies a different meaning. For example, a *period* in history is a particular and circumscribed length of time in which certain significant events occurred; but a *period* in grammar is a mark of punctuation. The two contexts lend different shades of meaning to the same concept. By looking closely at the various uses of *period,* however, you can determine that there are some essential elements that remain constant over all contexts, such as the element of an end point. Wilson points out that it is the sensitivity of the analyst to these *essential* and *nonessential* elements that makes for a successful analysis. In all concept analyses, the goal is clarity of language and cogency of communication. Therefore, determining the really essential or typical features of a concept is a priority.

In the case of *science,* many definitions have been formulated over time. In the interests of brevity, only the most common ones will be used here.

Webster's New Universal Unabridged Dictionary (1983) defines science as

a) state or fact of knowing; knowledge; b) systematized knowledge derived from observation, study, and experimentation carried on in order to determine the nature or principles of what is being studied; c) a branch of knowledge or study, especially one concerned with establishing and systematizing facts, principles, and methods, as by experiments and hypotheses; d) the systematized knowledge of nature and the physical world; e) skill, technique, or ability based upon training, discipline, and experience.

Shapere (1984), a sociologist of science, defined science as the "process by which areas or fields of scientific investigation are formed." Woolgar (1988), also a sociologist of science, stated that "what counts as science varies according to the particular textual purposes for which this is an issue." In effect, he argues that science is basically a social activity engaged in by participants who define science within the context of their interactions. Griffin (1988), a philosopher of science, defined science as "the attempt to establish truth through demonstrations open to experiential replication" (p. 26).

Model Cases

One of the best ways to begin a good analysis is to find an instance that the investigator is absolutely sure is an example of the concept under study. The instance should be so obvious that you could say, "Well if *that* isn't an example of so-and-so, then nothing is" (Wilson, 1963, p. 28). The model case is used to help the analyst see what the essential features are that allow a person to use the word correctly. Model cases are the paradigm, or exemplary, cases of the concept under study. Therefore they are critical to a good analysis. Most model cases are chosen based on the analyst's working definition of the concept. Moreover, the development of the model case is iterative; that is, the analyst works back and forth between the various cases and the working definition until the essential features of the concept become clear.

Wilson also suggested using more than one model case and comparing them. In this way, he said, the analyst can compare the essential features of each to see which ones are present in all cases. These would then be the essential features of the concept. Wilson warned, though, that some concepts do not have critical or essential features but do have typical features. That is, there may be concepts that have no single feature in common but that are linked by a group of characteristics. He gave the example of the concept of *games*, in which a typical feature is that two or more people can play. Yet it is not an essential feature since there are games like solitaire that do not require two people and that still clearly count as games.

In the example of science, a model case might be one such as this: A chemist is running a series of experiments in the laboratory. Based on previous work in the field, the chemist hypothesizes that a particular combination of chemicals will produce a drug that will reduce blood pressure in experimental rats. Over time, the chemist tries many combinations and amounts of the chemicals until a set is found that does reduce blood pressure in the rats. After many trials with that combination of chemicals, the chemist publishes an article in a refereed journal reporting the findings of the studies, linking them to other studies that have been done previously, proposing some changes in the underlying theory, and suggesting areas for further study.

Another case might be that of a nurse, who in the course of practice, observes certain recurring behaviors in a particular set of patients with a particular nursing diagnosis. On the basis of both literature review and clinical judgement, the nurse sets up a series of experimental therapies using volunteers from among the patients with the relevant diagnosis. Analysis of the data leads the nurse to believe that one treatment is substantially better than the others in outcomes. After publishing the initial results, the nurse conducts several more studies to confirm the findings. Finally, the nurse writes a theoretical paper synthesizing the results of all the studies and proposes a therapeutic model for the treatment of the particular diagnosis.

These are cases easily recognized by people as examples of *science*. What are the distinguishing characteristics as seen in these two cases? The elements common to both cases are knowledge generation, knowledge testing, knowledge organization, and knowledge accumulation. There is also an element of experience involved, as both scientists are skilled practitioners. In addition, both scientists communicated their work to others in their respective disciplines, and both were concerned with real world problems. That is, each scientist expects his or her work to have some practical significance in the future. There is a sense of ongoing activity as well.

Contrary Cases

The opposite method can also be helpful. That is, one can find an instance in which one could say "Well, whatever so-and-so is, *that* certainly isn't an instance of it" (Wilson, 1963, p. 29). Again, Wilson suggested using more than one contrary case, if necessary, and comparing across cases to discover what it is about them that makes them cases of **not**-the-concept. The features of the cases that make them contrary furnish clues to what features might be essential to the concept under study.

In the case of science, a contrary case is the following: a mother is watching her twins play in the back yard with a friend. She observes that the twins behave differently with one another than with their friend. She does not understand why this is so. After watching for a few moments, she turns away and begins washing the dishes.

This is clearly not an instance of science. The mother makes observations, but there is no effort to interpret them, to study the phenomenon systematically, or to accumulate or communicate the knowledge in any way.

Related Cases

Most concepts are not studied in isolation. As a rule, the concept under study is connected to other concepts that are similar or that occur in similar contexts. One must examine the network of concepts of which the concept under study is a part in order to truly understand how the study concept is the same and how it is different from those in the same network with it. It is through the critical examination of the network of related concepts that the analyst can gain insight into what features of the study concept are essential and which are not.

For the concept of science, *philosophy* is a related concept, as is *scholarship.* In *philosophy* the case might be that of a professor writing a series of treatises on the origins of ethical reasoning in the Celtic culture. For *scholarship* the case might be that of a student carefully examining all the literature on a given topic and writing a paper synthesizing the knowledge.

Neither of these cases is an example of science, although they are closer to it than the contrary case. Both are cases of scholarly endeavor, but they do not encompass all the essential elements of science. In the case of philosophy, there is no knowledge testing and no evidence in the case that the professor has plans to share the treatises with his professional colleagues. Nor is there evidence that the activity will be ongoing. In the scholarship case the student is synthesizing accumulated knowledge but is not generating it, testing it, or sharing it. Nor is the student likely to continue with the activity once the paper is turned in!

Borderline Cases

Borderline cases are those in which the analyst is not sure whether a case fits as an example of the concept or not. The analyst deliberately uses instances that are difficult to classify. By understanding what makes them difficult to classify, the analyst can often determine which elements are essential to the concept and which are not. This activity helps the analyst clarify what counts as the concept and what does not.

In the case of science, one borderline case might be a single study and another might be, for example, a car mechanic searching for the solution to a problem until it is found. In a study, hypotheses are generated and tested and results are obtained. The difference between science and a single study is that a single study can either generate knowledge or test knowledge, but unless that knowledge is published it does not add to a body of knowledge. The researcher may or may not be skilled and the research may or may not be concerned with a real world problem. A single research study does not imply any ongoing work. Research is only a method of science, it is not science itself. The case of the car mechanic is also a borderline case as hypotheses are tested until a solution is found. Moreover, no knowledge may be generated, no additions are made to the body of knowledge of the field, and the mechanic may or may not be skilled in his or her practice.

Invented Cases

Sometimes, the concept under study is such that the scientist cannot discover a sufficient number of different instances to clarify the concept. In this case, it is often helpful to take the concept outside of one's own experience. Wilson (1963) used the concept of "man" to illustrate his point (p. 32). Finding the essential criteria for a man is particularly difficult when in our world men are so easily classified as *men*. This may seem confusing since it suggests that one might need to invent cases when concepts are rare and also when concepts are very familiar. This is, however, exactly what Wilson meant. It is not the rarity of the concept or its frequency but the generalized agreement across cultures about what counts as the concept that is problematic.

To determine what the essential elements of *man* are, since there is such universal agreement across cultures about what a *man* is, one cannot find enough different instances of it to clarify the concept. Wilson suggested that taking a concept out of its context and using our imagination to understand our actual experience is often a fruitful way to grasp the essential elements of the concept under study. For instance, Wilson asked whether a creature who lives on the earth, has intelligence, and looks like a man but has no emotions, no art, and no sense of humor would count as a man. Since we identified relatively clear cases for the concept of science, no invented case was developed.

Social Context

Language only occurs within a social context. Thus, concepts take on meaning within that social context. But, social contexts differ across cultures, across regions, and even across disciplines. Therefore, the sensitive analyst must take into account the social milieu in which the concept under study is used. The analyst might ask who might use the concept, when it might be used, why it might be used, and so forth as a way of determining the context in which it is likely to be used.

There seems to be more controversy over how *science* is defined than over the context in which it occurs. Most discussions of the term seem to hold to the view that science occurs in laboratories, in academic sites, in industry and commerce, and in clinical settings. Nevertheless, there may be subtle variations in the conceptual context even when there is general agreement about where it occurs. For instance, a chemist in an industrial setting might see science somewhat differently from a social worker in a family abuse shelter. Although the essential elements of science remain the same, the foci of the two disciplines may be such that what is seen as "good" science may be somewhat different. The choices of research methods may be different, or the emphasis on the individual essential elements may have different weights.

Underlying Anxiety

Associated with the idea of a social context for concepts is the idea that most persons use concepts for a purpose. That is, there is an underlying feeling or tone with all use of language. If the analyst can determine what feelings might be associated with the concept under study, some important insights about the concept may emerge. For instance, the analyst might ask, Has the concept generated strong feelings or controversy? Is there debate about the issue? Is it generally positive, or is it negative?

In nursing, the underlying anxiety about *science* seems to be a need to justify the discipline's existence and make it a legitimate academic enterprise. Interestingly, this is true not only of nursing but of other young sciences such as sociology and social work as well. There seems to be a feeling in the young disciplines that until the discipline achieves *science,* it is not valid. Moreover, in many of the young sciences the methods of the more established natural sciences are not always useful. The newer disciplines are working, along with nursing, to find better ways to acquire and accumulate knowledge; the analysts in these fields are thereby shaping and refining their understanding of the concept of science.

Practical Results

Wilson said that understanding a concept ought to make some difference in our lives. In other words, there ought to be some practical result from understanding the essential elements of a concept. If there is no practical result from analysis of a concept, then something is seriously amiss with the language in which the question of concept was put. He suggests that if we understand the concept, we are more likely to understand the underlying worries of the person who is using it. And by understanding the underlying worries we are more likely to respond to those worries appropriately.

In terms of the example concept with which we have been working, there seem to be four essential elements of the term *science.* The first is that science is concerned with knowledge—its generation, testing, organization, and accumulation. The second is that science is an experiential process that involves highly developed skills. The third is that science is a social activity within a group of like-minded scholars. The fourth is that there is some concern for truth in science; that is, the scientist is interested in at least some relationship between the knowledge developed and the world as it is experienced day by day.

Results in Language

The final step in Wilson's procedure for concept analysis is obtaining results in language. Since words often have ambiguous meanings, it is not always possible to be decisive about *the* single or central meaning of a word. It is, however, still sensible to adopt one meaning over another. The purpose in doing so is to find the one meaning that works most efficiently, but that is not so restricted that it ceases to have any function at all. In other words, Wilson suggested that when one is choosing the essential features of a concept, one should choose those that are most useful. Wilson (1963) said that after careful concept analysis, one should be able to say, "Amid all these possible meanings of the word so-and-so, it seems most sensible and useful to make it mean such-and-such: for in this way we shall be able to use the word to its fullest advantage" (p. 37).

For the concept of *science,* the following is the most useful definition: the knowledge seeking, knowledge acquiring, knowledge accumulating, knowledge organizing, and knowledge disseminating activities of scholars in a particular field. These activities require a significant degree of skill, are experientially based, and are expected to produce knowledge that relates in some way with the world as it is experienced.

Conclusion

The Wilson (1963) method of concept analysis is an effective, easy-to-use method for discovering the essential features of a concept. Although it often seems a lengthy process to novices, it can be a helpful strategy, particularly in cases in which the concept is vague or has more than one meaning. His method is not complex and can be accomplished by persons as young as teenagers. It is an extremely useful strategy for classroom use in small groups and as a way of stimulating lively discussions. It is also very helpful for novice researchers as they attempt to arrive at operational definitions for their variables of interest.

Wilson suggested that the best way to conduct a good concept analysis is to follow all the steps in order. Yet he admitted that in some cases one or more of the last four steps may be either too obvious or irrelevant. In analyses where that is so, the irrelevant steps may be omitted. The sensitivity of the analyst will enable her or him to make good use of the appropriate steps of the strategy.

In nursing, one of the most important tasks facing us as we develop our own science is the naming and development of our concepts. Until we have identified our concepts of concern, our science will not grow very rapidly. Concept analysis is extremely useful as a tool for clarifying potential concepts of interest.

Concept analysis is also valuable prior to tool development. Nursing lacks appropriate tools to measure many important concepts. A good concept analysis yields essential elements of the concept that can then be incorporated into tools for measuring the concept. And when a tool is developed using concept analysis as a base, the researcher already has a head start on construct validity.

There are limits to what concept analysis can do, however. It cannot generate new concepts. It cannot give answers to all our questions about what concepts should have the most emphasis in the discipline, nor can it tell us which concepts are the best for nursing.

A single concept, by itself, is only useful for naming a phenomenon. But when it is related to other concepts, it becomes more useful to the discipline. Concepts in relationships or patterns are what drive nurse scholars to ask questions, to try to answer those questions, and to contribute to the development of nursing *science.*

REFERENCES

Griffin, D. R. (1988). *The reenchantment of science.* New York: State University of New York.
Shapere, D. (1984). *Reason and the search for knowledge.* Boston: D. Reidel.
Webster, N. (1983). *Webster's new universal unabridged dictionary* (2nd ed.). New York: Dorset & Baber.
Wilson, J. (1963). *Thinking with concepts.* Cambridge: Cambridge University Press.
Woolgar, S. (1988). *Science: The very idea.* New York: Tavistock.

Chapter 5

Wilsonian Concept Analysis: Applying the Technique

KAY C. AVANT AND CYNTHIA ALLEN ABBOTT

*I*n this chapter the technique suggested by Wilson (1963) will be
used to examine a concept relevant to nursing practice. We have chosen
the concept of delegation for analysis. It is abstract enough to lend itself to
analysis; it is relevant to nursing practice; and it may have several different
meanings. Since nurses are involved in delegation in all aspects of their
work, a clear understanding of the essential elements of delegation is appropriate.

This chapter is organized around Wilson's (1963) eleven steps as described in chapter 4. The reader is referred to chapter 4 for a full explanation
of each of the steps.

Isolating Questions of Concept

Questions are often raised about the nature of delegation and nursing care.
Certain questions may be at issue, such as, Should nursing care ever be
delegated? If a situation calls for delegation, is there ever one in which the
authority is delegated but the responsibility is not? and To whom is it
appropriate to delegate certain nursing care? However, these are not pure
questions of concept. The first question is a question of value. It calls for
both an analysis of the concept of delegation and a value judgment about
its use. The second question is also a mixed question. It calls for a concept
analysis for three different concepts (delegation, authority, and responsibility) and also for a policy analysis of the appropriate use of the concepts
analyzed. The third question calls for a concept analysis and also is a question
requiring the use of facts about the nature and qualifications of those to
whom the delegated action might be given. A true question of concept
would be, What is the logical nature of the concept of delegation? Therefore,

These are the views of the author (Cynthia Abbott) and do not represent the views of the
U.S. Army, Department of Defense.

it is the answer to this last question which this concept analysis will attempt
to provide.

Right Answers

Wilson (1963) pointed out that there are no final right answers in a concept
analysis. However, he did emphasize that there are primary and central uses
for concepts that can be distinguished by a thoughtful analysis. The effort
is to determine which elements of the concept of delegation are the important or essential ones and which ones are extensions, derivations, or
metaphors of the concept.

The concept of delegation has two principal uses. The first has to do
with the act of assigning. The second use refers to a group with a mission.

In the first case the process of delegation includes ideas such as supervision and assignment of duties, the transfer of authority or accountability
to subordinates for completion of work, and use of time and expertise
effectively (Rees, 1988). Delegation also includes the ideas of authority,
communication, responsibility, monitoring, and work. To maximize the
chances of delegation's producing a successful outcome, the superior must
assess the subordinate (Keenan, Hurst, Dennis, & Frey, 1990; McAlvanah,
1989; McConkey, 1986; Poteet, 1984; Rees, 1988), the complexity of the
work or task to be done (American Association of Critical Care Nurses
[AACN], 1990; Bentley, 1985; Harbin, 1990; Keenan, Hurst, Dennis & Frey,
1990; McAlvanah, 1989; McConkey, 1986; Murphy, 1984; Olivant, 1984;
Poteet, 1984, 1986), and the context or situation in which the work is to
be done (AACN, 1990; Bass, Valenzi, Farrow, & Solomon, 1975; Blau &
Scott, 1962; Hoy & Bousa, 1984; Leana, 1986, 1987; Runnie, 1985; Vinton,
1987) before making the assignment.

The superior assigns the subordinate to complete a specific task (AACN,
1990; Anders, 1988; Anderson, 1984, Haynes, 1974; Hoy & Bousa, 1984;
Leana, 1986; Poteet, 1984, 1986; Rees, 1988; Vinton, 1987). The superior
communicates to the subordinate (Bass, Valenzi, Farrow, & Solomon, 1975;
Harbin, 1990; McAlvanah, 1989; Olivant, 1984; Poteet, 1984; Runnie, 1985;
Shapira, 1976; Vinton, 1987; Watson, 1983) the needed performance criteria
(Harbin, 1990; McConkey, 1986; Poteet, 1984; Rees, 1988; Watson, 1983),
time allowed (Poteet, 1986), and plans for providing feedback (AACN, 1990;
Bentley, 1985; Keenan, Hurst, Dennis, & Frey, 1990; Rees, 1988). The su-
perior transfers to the subordinate the authority (AACN, 1990; Anderson,
1984; Hoy & Bousa, 1984; Leana, 1986, 1987; Murphy, 1984; Rees, 1988;
Runnie, 1985; Shapira, 1976; Vinton, 1987), resources (Bentley, 1985;
Haynes, 1974; Rees, 1988; Vinton, 1987), and responsibility necessary to
complete the task or work (Anders, 1988; Anderson, 1984; Bentley, 1985;
Haynes, 1974; Keenan, Hurst, Dennis, & Frey, 1990; McAlvanah, 1989;

McConkey, 1986; Murphy, 1984; Poteet, 1986; Rees, 1988; Simpson & Sears, 1985). The superior does not interfere with task completion unless assistance is sought by the subordinate (Hoy & Bousa, 1984; Keenan, Hurst, Dennis, & Frey, 1990; Leana, 1986, 1987; Rees, 1988; Simpson & Sears, 1985; Vinton, 1987). The superior completes the work through the subordinate (Drucker, 1963).

In the second case the person (delegate) is selected, elected, or appointed by another person, a group of persons, or an organization to represent their interests, usually to an even larger body of persons or organizations. A set of such selected persons is referred to as a *delegation*. The delegation here is a body of people and is not the activity itself. This second use of the concept delegation appears to be an extension of the primary concept in that the delegates are the ones who receive the assignment. The real delegation occurs from the group or organization that selects or appoints the delegates. Therefore, it is the first use of the concept that will be considered here since it is the primary concept, or the activity of delegation, that is of interest to us.

Model Cases

Case 1. A working mother is feeling overwhelmed with all the tasks she must accomplish in two hours to prepare for a dinner party for six close friends. She considers ways to decrease the number of things she must do. She reviews which tasks are most complicated and decides that only she can plan the menu and prepare the meal for the dinner party. Two other tasks are vacuuming the carpets and dusting the furniture. She believes her ten-year-old daughter can vacuum and dust reliably since the daughter has done these chores several times before under the mother's supervision.

The mother directs the daughter to vacuum the carpets and dust before 6 PM. She needs to vacuum the hall, living room, and dining room to remove the visible dirt and lint on the floors. She does not need to vacuum behind the furniture. She should dust the furniture in those same three rooms. The mother tells the daughter she is to ask her if more information or assistance is needed in doing the task.

As the daughter vacuums, the father comes down the hall in muddy shoes. The daughter cries out, "Stop, you have to take your shoes off! I'm cleaning the floor for mom and I don't want to vacuum the hall again!" The father does as the daughter says and takes off his shoes before continuing down the hall. The mother occasionally checks the progress and quality of vacuuming and dusting completed. Finally, the mother examines the completed job, provides approval of the work, and rewards the daughter by allowing her to have a friend over the next night to play.

Case 2. A second model case, taken from nursing, is the case of the nursing team leader making assignments for the upcoming shift. She reviews the case load, the patient acuity status, and the number and type of staff she will have on duty. She knows that several of the patients are very sick and will need her best staff nurses. A number of patients are not so sick and will need less skilled care. When her staff arrives, she discusses the case load with them and assigns the care of specific patients according to her knowledge of the skill levels of the staff and the needs of the patients. She tells staff members what her expectations are and tells them to ask for help if they need it.

Later in the morning, as she makes rounds to check on the patients and the staff, the new staff nurse asks for help calibrating an infusion pump. The team leader shows the nurse how to calibrate the pump, then watches as the nurse calibrates the infusion properly. She commends the new nurse on his skill and on his willingness to ask for help.

Conclusions. In both of these cases, there are common elements. In each case there is work to be done, a person who is responsible for the work to be done (superior or delegator), and another person to whom the work is assigned (subordinate or delegate). In each case the delegator communicates what work is to be done and her expectations for the completion of the work. Access to needed resources is provided to the delegate. The delegator monitors the progress of the work and rewards the delegate at the successful completion of the work. The delegate in each case assumes responsibility for performing the work, demonstrates the authority or ability to carry it out, and completes the work.

Contrary Cases

Contrary cases are those cases that clearly do not apply to the concept under study. Contrary cases help to clarify the essential elements of the concept by focusing on the opposite of it. Sometimes it is easier to say what a thing is not, than to say what it is. The contrary cases give a different view of the concept and allow the analyst to compare one case against its opposite.

Case 1. A contrary case from the model case might be that of a working mother who is feeling overwhelmed with all the tasks she must accomplish in two hours to prepare for a dinner party for six close friends. She goes over the tasks and prioritizes them. She decides to dust the furniture but not to vacuum, to clean the bathroom but not the bedrooms, and to simplify the menu by purchasing dessert instead of making it herself. She picks up the dessert on the way home from work. When she gets home, she hastily completes all the tasks she has listed and with dinner in the oven, finds she has just enough time to change her clothes before the guests arrive.

Case 2. A contrary case in nursing might be that of Mr. Smith, one of two team leaders on his unit. Mr. Smith walks through a bad snow storm to get to work one morning only to discover that he is the only one on his team who has managed to get to work so far. There are messages from three others on the team that they are on their way but that they are delayed because of unplowed streets. He calls the nursing supervisor to report his plight, but she tells him he is not alone. The same situation has happened all over the hospital. She tells him that she has asked some night staff to stay on for at least another hour or so and that she has called an agency for help. In the meantime, he must just do the best he can until she can send him some help. Sighing, Mr. Smith reviews the patient load, prioritizes the tasks to be done, and taking the highest priorities first, begins to work. He continues to complete the high priority tasks as best he can and hopes fervently for more help to arrive soon.

Conclusions. These cases are not cases of delegation. Although the woman has a lot of work to do, she never seeks to assign any of it to anyone else. She does review the tasks and determines priorities, but she never communicates them to anyone and does not ask for help. Mr. Smith also does not delegate. He does review the tasks and assigns priorities. If more of his team arrives later, he will delegate some of the work at that point. However, since he is alone, he cannot delegate.

Related Cases

Related cases are cases that somehow are similar to or connected with the concept under analysis. In the case of the concept of delegation, the concepts of trust and of referring and transferring seemed to be the most germane since delegation is often difficult when trust has not been established between the delegator and the delegate and since referring and transferring are often used as synonyms for delegation. Distinguishing among these concepts should aid the analysis of delegation.

Case 1. Jonathon is the commander of a garrison on the frontier. His scout, David, tells him there are enemy troops just over the hill from the garrison headquarters. Although Jonathon does not see the enemy soldiers, he calls his officers together and tells them to prepare for a possible enemy attack. His officers question why he is preparing for attack when no enemy is in sight. He replies, "I trust David's report."

Conclusion. The concept of trust is defined in *Webster's Ninth New Collegiate Dictionary* as "assured reliance on the character, ability, strength, or truth of someone or something" (1983). It involves a relationship between two persons in which one can be confident of the other's abilities and values and can depend on the other to behave in certain ways under certain conditions. Trust between a superior and a subordinate is antecedent to delegation since the delegator must be confident of the delegate before giving him or her the assignment.

Case 2. Mrs. Lorenson, the high school counselor, is called to the teacher's lounge by Mr. Clark, the math teacher. When she arrives, she finds Mr. Clark and Dorothy, a junior student. Dorothy is crying, wringing her hands, and looking fearfully toward the corner of the room. Mr. Clark tells Mrs. Lorenson that Dorothy began acting strangely in class, mumbling at first and then yelling "Get away from me! Get away!" even though no one was near her at the time. Mr. Clark says, "I am not equipped to handle this one. I will leave her in your capable hands." He leaves the room and returns to class.

Conclusion. The concept of referring is sometimes used as a synonym for delegation. To refer is to "think of, regard, or classify within a general category or group; to send or direct for treatment, aid, information or decision" (*Webster's,* 1983). From the case and from the definition it can be seen that to refer something involves giving up the decision-making task altogether. The person making the referral may not retain any of the responsibility for further decision making once the referral is made. The referring individual does not communicate how the job is to be done, does not provide resources to do the job, and does not monitor the results.

Case 3. Mrs. Lorenson attempts to talk to Dorothy but is unable to get her to respond. After several attempts she takes Dorothy to her office and calls Dorothy's parents. She explains the situation to the parents and tells them that they must come and pick Dorothy up. She explains that the school system is not prepared to deal with such a situation. When the parents arrive, Mrs. Lorenson urges them to seek immediate treatment for Dorothy and provides the names of several psychologists who treat teenagers. She hands Dorothy over to them and sadly watches as the family leaves the school.

Conclusion. The concept of transferring is also related to delegation. It is defined as "to convey from one person, place, or situation to another; to cause to pass from one to another" (*Webster's,* 1983). In the case of transfer, the person transferring again retains no authority or responsibility for the item or work that is passed to the other. Little or no communication about the item or work may take place between the transferring person and the person to whom the item or work is transferred.

Borderline Cases

Borderline cases are those in which one is not sure whether the case is one of delegation. The borderline cases are particularly useful because by trying to see what makes them borderline, it is possible to determine what there is in the model case that is essential. Two borderline cases are used in this analysis to point out essential features of delegation.

Case 1. The high school needed a significant curriculum change. The principal was asked by a group of faculty to consider a revised curriculum. The principal formed a task force of teachers to consider all areas of possible change such as content areas, recommended textbooks, teaching styles, and ancillary support required to implement a new curriculum. She gave the task force access to all needed resources and gave the members authority to ask other faculty for additional information. The principal gave the task force performance criteria, time expectations, and planned weekly meetings to guide job completion. She stated that if the aforementioned criteria were met and if the faculty reached 100 percent agreement on all aspects of the proposed curriculum, the group would be able to implement the proposed curriculum as a pilot program. During weekly meetings the principal insisted that the task force make significant changes in their ideas and plans. Within the allotted time the task force completed the formal proposal with required criteria and support of all faculty. The principal did allow the faculty to implement the proposed curriculum as a pilot program.

Conclusion. The critical attributes of assignment, communication, and reward are present, but the attribute of transfer of authority is altered. Although access to needed resources was given, the principal did not allow the task force to complete the assignment without interference in their decision making. Her need to direct the task force when not asked interfered with the transference of authority to subordinates.

Case 2. Julia is a new head nurse who is trying to introduce a more participatory management style on her unit. Therefore, upon reviewing the case load and acuity level of patients and finding that most of the patients were no longer critical, she decides to let her staff make the assignments as a group after shift report. When the shift report is finished, she asks the staff, "Now, how are we going to arrange it so all these patients get the best care we can give them?" The staff sit down together, discuss the needs of each patient, and decide as a group who will take care of each one. The head nurse is pleased with the resulting decisions and smiles to herself as the staff leave discussing how pleased they are with their work assignments.

Conclusion. This case is also a borderline case. Some of the essential elements of the model case are present, but some are not. There is work to be done. There is a superior and a group of subordinates, but they are not treated strictly as subordinates by the superior. Assignments are made but not by the superior. There is communication about the work to be done and expectations about how it should be done, but both are defined by the group and not by the superior. The superior does monitor the proceedings but does not interfere. The staff assume responsibility for the work and carry it out.

Invented Cases

Invented cases are used when the concept under study does not provide a sufficient number of instances of the concept to clarify it (Wilson, 1963). In the case of delegation there are numerous instances, and an invented case is not strictly necessary. However, for the purposes of demonstrating the application of all of the steps in Wilson's (1963) method, an invented case has been included here.

Case Study. The king rat on planet Noah was a biblical historian and an astrologer. Wise men of his planet had predicted since his birth that his reign as king would end in the destruction of the planet. The king rat realized the predictions would soon be true, for in two months the planet Noah would collide with the sun. However, he had a plan to save the various species on the planet, based on knowledge of biblical literature.

The king rat devised a master plan and called his most trusted experts to meet. He charged the experts, such as anthropologists, sociologists, biologists, and nurse scientists, to choose one male and one female of fertile age from each species on the planet to represent inhabitants of the planet. He set the day the selection was to be complete and told the experts to use his name if anyone obstructed their mission. He proclaimed all of the experts to have supreme access to needed transportation, food, housing, staff, and any additional support requested. Additionally, he commissioned the air force high command to ready a spaceship with sufficient supplies and adequate environmental conditions to sustain all life for three years or until a safe haven was identified. The planet earth was deemed a possible haven since it had reportedly undergone a similar crisis with floods light years ago.

The king rat made it clear that he was available for counsel. He stated that he would oversee the results of the plan as experts progressed in their mission. Each expert was expected to contact him if problems that interfered with progress were encountered. Additionally, he reminded each member of the seriousness of the mission and of the potential consequences for the future life on planet Noah if even one individual did not succeed in effectively completing the collection of the species. At the completion of the mission and departure of the space ship from the planet Noah, the king rat praised the experts in public and knighted them for their success in completing the mission.

Conclusion. A superior-subordinate relationship involving trust and subordinate expertise is seen between the king and his subordinates. Additionally, this case illustrates the planning the king rat completed before assigning missions and charging the experts. Once assignments were made, the king transferred the authority to the experts by allowing them to use his name if they encountered resistance. Monitoring was addressed by supervising the progress of results as they occurred incrementally. Expecting the subordinate to tell the king if problems interfered with progress implies a transfer of responsibility for progress of the mission. Additionally, reviewing the consequences for the entire project should a mission fail transferred a piece of responsibility for the mission success to each subordinate. Access to all resources to include additional staff was transferred. And finally, the subordinates were rewarded for their work.

Social Context

The social context in which a concept is used can provide the analyst with insight into the essential nature of the concept. For instance, the concept of delegation is most often used in the context of business and management. Persons in positions of authority, and often those in subordinate positions as well, may be concerned about the proper use of delegation. When it is appropriate and when it is not, to whom tasks can or should be delegated, and how much monitoring is sufficient for delegated tasks are recurrent issues. Nurses are concerned with delegation at all levels. Nurse managers delegate to staff; staff delegate to assistive personnel; and, of course, physicians delegate to nurses as well. The complexity of the social contexts of health care agencies and systems, when considered alongside the social mandate for nurses to provide the best quality care in the most efficient and effective manner, makes delegation a critical issue. To understand the concept of delegation, one must understand the complex nature of the health care system in which it occurs and the moral, legal, and technical issues surrounding delegation in that context.

The aspects of delegation most reflected in the social context have to do with the superior's assessment of the tasks to be done, the prioritizing of those tasks, the abilities of the subordinates, and the trust she or he has in those subordinates. In a system as complex as a health care agency, it is no small responsibility the superior holds in making those decisions. If the superior is new to the system, for instance, or is inexperienced as a supervisor, the quality of this assessment may suffer. As a consequence of poor assessment, tasks may be delegated inappropriately, leading to inefficient, ineffective care. On the whole, inappropriate delegation may result in poor patient care.

Underlying Anxiety

Closely associated with considering the social context of a concept is examining the underlying anxiety associated with it. It seems to us that there are at least two underlying anxieties associated with the concept of delegation. First is the issue of whether any nursing task ought to be delegated at all. If a task is a nursing task, should it not be performed by a nurse? And yet, there are too many tasks and not enough nurses to carry them all out. Management decisions regarding hospital staffing levels may require that nurses delegate many tasks to nonnurses in order that patients receive adequate care.

A second underlying source of anxiety is what nursing tasks are safe to delegate and to whom? Does the context in which the tasks are to take place make a difference in whether they can be delegated? For instance, delegating the bath and linen change for a patient who is recovering from elective surgery and ready for discharge on the following day is potentially different from delegating the bath and linen change for a newly admitted, critically ill patient in medical intensive care. The issue of trust in the superior-subordinate relationship is important in resolving the underlying anxieties associated with delegation.

Both the social context and the underlying anxiety of the concept of delegation demonstrate that the issue of complexity of task, superior-subordinate trust, and ability of the delegate are important aspects of delegation. It must be the responsibility of the delegator or supervisor to clearly understand the task and the person delegated to perform the task.

Practical Results

Wilson (1963) pointed out quite accurately that analyzing a concept should have some practical results. That is, one should consider what the purpose is in analyzing a concept. If the results are not useful, analyzing the concept is a waste of time. In the case of the concept of delegation, we feel that understanding the logical structure of the concept will help us to teach nurses what delegation entails and will also help us measure the concept in research. An understanding of the logical structure of the concept will provide a frame of reference for our work.

Results in Language

Wilson (1963) suggested that in defining a logical structure for a concept one should take care to choose the most useful criteria for the concept of interest. That is, care must be taken not to delimit the concept so much that it is essentially banned from one's working vocabulary. On the other hand, the concept should not be so loosely limited that it can be used in almost any situation and thus, in effect, becomes meaningless. Therefore, the priority of the analyst of any concept should be to choose the critical elements in such a way as to allow the use of the concept to its fullest advantage.

Conclusions

Having progressed through Wilson's eleven steps, we can now examine the results of our analysis to determine the logical structure of the concept of delegation. The premier consideration of an analysis, for Wilson, is the identification of the essential elements of the concept under analysis. Therefore, as a result of our analysis, the essential elements of the concept of delegation are as follows:

1. There must be a superior-subordinate relationship in which the superior has both responsibility and authority.
2. There must be a level of trust between the superior (the delegator) and the subordinate (the delegate).
3. There must be a task or set of tasks to be accomplished.
4. The delegator must assess the situation in terms of the complexity, priority, and potential risks of the task as well as the abilities of the delegate.
5. The delegator must assign the task to the delegate.
6. The delegator must communicate to the delegate any expectations about the way the task is to be completed.
7. The delegator must provide the delegate with access to resources needed to complete the task.
8. The delegate must assume responsibility for the task.
9. The delegator must monitor the completion of the task and provide feedback to the delegate about the effectiveness of task completion.
10. Both delegator and delegate benefit from the experience.

From this list of essential elements or characteristics, a clear picture of the process of delegation appears. It would be possible, using this list of essential elements, to prepare a lesson plan to teach the process of delegation to beginners in management, to construct an evaluation instrument for assessing delegation, or to design a research tool by which one might measure delegation. To Wilson, the process of concept analysis is undertaken to clarify one's thinking and to make communication easier. This concept analysis of delegation has served that purpose for us. We hope it will serve the same purpose for our readers.

REFERENCES

American Association of Critical Care Nurses (AACN). (1990). *Delegation of nursing and nonnursing activities in critical care.* Laguna Nigual, Calif: AACN.

Anders, G.T. (August 15, 1988). Duties you should—and shouldn't—delegate. *Medical Economics,* pp. 182–191.

Anderson, J.G. (1984). When leaders develop themselves. *Training and Development Journal, 38*(6), 18–22.

Bass, B.M., Valenzi, E.R., Farrow, D.L., & Solomon, R.J. (1975). Management styles associated with organizational, task, personal, and interpersonal contingencies. *Journal of Applied Psychology, 60*(6), 720–729.

Bentley, C. (1985). All through the night. *Australian Nurses Journal, 14*(10), 41–44.

Blau, P.M., & Scott, W.R. (1962). *Formal Organizations.* New York: Chandler.

Drucker, P. (1963). Managing for business effectiveness. *Harvard Business Review, 41*(3), 18–26.

Harbin, R.E. (1990). Practicing effective delegation. *Pediatric Nursing, 16*(1), 91–92.

Haynes, M.E. (1974). Delegation: Key to involvement. *Personnel Journal, 53,* 454–456.

Hoy, W.K., & Bousa, D.A. (1984). Delegation: The neglected aspect of participation in decision making. *The Alberta Journal of Educational Research, 30,* 320–331.

Keenan, M.J., Hurst, J.B., Dennis, R.S., & Frey, G. (1990). Situational leadership for collaboration in health care settings. *Health Care Supervisor, 8*(3), 19–25.

Leana, C.R. (1986). Predictors and consequences of delegation. *Academy of Management Journal, 29,* 754–774.

Leana, C.R. (1987). Power relinquishment versus power sharing: Theoretical clarification and empirical comparison of delegation and participation. *Journal of Applied Psychology, 72,* 228–233.

McAlvanah, M.E. (1989). A guide to delegation. *Pediatric Nursing, 16,* 379.

McConkey, D.D. (1986). *No-nonsense delegation.* (rev. ed.). New York: American Management Association.

Murphy, E.C. (1984). Delegation—from denial to acceptance. *Nursing Management, 15*(1), 54–56.

Olivant, M. (1984). Delegation problems. *Nursing Times, 80*(31), 43–44.

Poteet, G.W. (1984). Delegation strategies a must for the nurse executive. *Journal of Nursing Administration, 14*(9), 18–21.

Poteet, G.W. (1986). Delegation strategies for the pediatric nurse. *Journal of Pediatric Nursing, 1,* 271–273.

Rees, R. (1988). Delegation: A fundamental management process. *Education Canada, 28*(2), 26–32.

Runnie, R.J. (1985). School centered management: A matter of style. *School Business Affairs, 51*(4), 64–67.

Shapira, Z. (1976). A facet analysis of leadership styles. *Journal of Applied Psychology, 61*(2), 136–139.

Simpson, K., & Sears R. (1985). Authority and responsibility delegation predicts quality of care. *Journal of Advanced Nursing, 10,* 345–348.

Vinton, D. (1987). Delegation for employee development. *Training and Development Journal, 4*(1), 65–67.

Watson, C. (1983). Third-stage limits and delegation. *Nursing Mirror, 156*(18), 35.

Webster's ninth new collegiate dictionary. (1983). Frederick C. Mish (editor-in-chief). Springfield, Mass: Merriam-Webster.

Wilson, J. (1963). *Thinking with concepts.* Cambridge: Cambridge University Press.

Chapter 6

Concept Analysis: An Evolutionary View

BETH L. RODGERS

*H*istorically, popular views of concepts and concept analysis have been based on a philosophical position known as essentialism. The purpose of analysis has been to define the concept of interest in terms of its critical attributes or *essence*. This essence generally appears as a set of conditions both necessary and sufficient to delineate the domain and boundaries of the concept. Consistent with a position of essentialism, the concept in such analyses is viewed apart from its context or any relationship with other concepts. Reports of this type of inquiry give the impression that the concept is both universal (i.e., without contextual variation) and unchanging. In other words, the results reveal precisely what the concept *is*.

Recently, philosophical discussions of concepts have presented views in opposition to the essentialist position. The current tendency has been to consider concepts as dynamic, rather than static; "fuzzy," rather than finite, absolute, and "crystal clear"; context dependent, rather than universal; and as possessing some pragmatic utility rather than an inherent "truth" (Ryle, 1971; Toulmin, 1972; Wittgenstein, 1953/1968; see Chapter 2). Significantly, this contemporary view of concepts has gained considerable support from empirical research in the field of psychology (Barsalou & Medin, 1986; Fehr, 1988; McCloskey & Glucksberg, 1978; Smith & Medin, 1981). This position is compatible with the perspective generally accepted in nursing, which espouses a view of reality, and of human beings and related nursing phenomena, as constantly changing, comprised of numerous interrelated and overlapping elements, and interpretable only in regard to a multitude of contextual factors.

Unfortunately, researchers have not operationalized fully the implications of contemporary philosophical positions in actual methods of concept analysis. Adherence to essentialism has compromised the significance and utility of attempts to clarify and develop concepts in nursing. One alternative approach to concept analysis, which I refer to as the "evolutionary" view (Rodgers, 1989a, 1989c), is derived from contemporary philosophical thought and was designed to overcome some of the difficulties associated with traditional positions.

The Philosophical Basis of the Evolutionary View

The evolutionary approach to concepts represents the integration of views expressed primarily by Toulmin (1972) and Wittgenstein (1953/1968), although Price (1953) and Ryle (1971) also were influential. According to this approach, a concept is considered to be an "abstraction that is expressed in some form" (Rodgers, 1989a, p. 332). In other words, concepts are formed by the identification of characteristics common to a class of objects or phenomena and the abstraction and clustering of these characteristics, along with some means of expression (usually a word). Although concepts are individual and private in nature, the process of abstraction, clustering, and association of the concept with a word (or other means of expression) is influenced heavily by socialization and public interaction. Consequently, the development of a concept for a person takes place with guidance from the social context in which the person interacts and develops concepts. Toulmin (1972) discussed this process in relation to socialization within a discipline; yet his term "enculturation" is appropriate to describe this process regardless of the specific context in which it occurs.

The forms of expression that are acquired along with a concept enable an individual to share his or her concepts publicly with others. Although these forms typically are discursive or linguistic, there may be nondiscursive forms as well, for example, through various means of artistic expression. These expressions provide access to an individual's concepts and reflect the use of the concept. Consequently, they provide the basis for concept analysis. It is important to note that a concept is not merely the word or expression but the mental cluster that lies behind the word. Words are manifestations of concepts (Price, 1953), not the concepts themselves. Examination of the common use of a concept, through these expressions, provides a means to explore the underlying concept and to identify its attributes (definition).

Although many scholars view the process of defining concepts as important, in existing discussions relatively little attention has been given to the relationship between concepts and knowledge. In other words, what purposes do concepts serve in the general enterprise of knowledge development? According to Toulmin (1972), concepts, especially what he termed "scientific" concepts, contribute to knowledge because of their inherent "explanatory" powers. (A thorough reading of Toulmin's work reveals that he used the terms *scientific* and *explanatory* quite loosely. Nonetheless, it is probably more appropriate to refer to concepts as having explanatory or descriptive power.) One of the primary functions of concepts is to facilitate categorizations. In other words, concepts are important in determining how to refer to or discuss certain situations, events, or phenomena, and how various conceptual categories may be related to each other. With clear concepts it is possible to "explain" phenomena as belonging to or indicative of a particular concept and, consequently, as possessing certain attributes. Ultimately, concepts can be used to characterize phenomena of interest, to describe situations, and to communicate effectively.

When the attributes (definition) that comprise the concept are unclear, the ability to communicate and categorize phenomena is severely limited. Analysis of the common use of the concept, by examining means of expression, enables the researcher to identify the cluster of attributes that constitute the concept and, hence, to define the concept. As a result, the concept may be used more effectively. With a clearly defined concept it is possible to classify or characterize phenomena more adequately and, in turn, to evaluate the strengths and limitations of the concept. Ultimately, variations can be introduced and tested, with the result being an even more useful concept and one that reflects a contemporary context for its use.

This process of definition, evaluation, and refinement is important in the development of knowledge. The goal is to clarify and develop concepts that are clear and useful. Most important, however, is the generation of concepts that resolve existing conceptual problems. This notion of development and refinement reveals the emphasis placed on conceptual change or *evolution* within this view of concepts. I do not consider the attributes of a concept to be a fixed set of necessary and sufficient conditions, or an *essence.* Consequently, according to this view, this cluster of attributes may change, by convention or by purposeful redefinition, over time to maintain a useful, applicable, and effective concept.

THE CONCEPT DEVELOPMENT CYCLE

The process of concept development can be presented as a cycle that continues through time and within a particular context (Figure 6–1). The context may be that of a particular discipline, cultural group, or, on some occasions, the context provided by a particular theory. Three distinct influences on concept development are apparent and include the significance, use, and application of the concept. The significance of the concept reflects Toulmin's (1972) observation that "concepts acquire a meaning through serving the relevant human purpose in actual practical cases" (p. 168). This "relevant purpose" is the concept's ability to resolve problems and to characterize phenomena adequately, thus furthering progress in the development of knowledge. As Toulmin indicated, the significance given to a par-

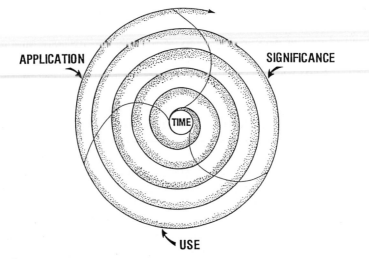

APPLICATION   SIGNIFICANCE

TIME

USE

Figure 6–1 Cycle of Concept Development
Reprinted with permission from B. L. Rodgers (1989). Concepts, analysis, and the development
of nursing knowledge: The evolutionary cycle. *Journal of Advanced Nursing, 14,* 330–335.

ticular concept at any point in time is related to a variety of factors. The
importance attached to a particular concept or conceptual problem, for
example, provides a strong incentive internal to a discipline to focus efforts
on the development of the concept. Other factors, referred to as external
because they lie beyond the boundaries of the particular discipline, include
various rewards and incentives to develop particular concepts. Overall, a
concept that is considered significant will be used often, emphasized, and
studied, all of which enhance the development of clearer and more useful
concepts (Rodgers, 1989a, 1989c).

Significance thus has a profound effect on the use of the concept. Use,
in this sense, refers to the common manner of employing the concept and
the situations appropriate for its use. Consistent with the definition of *concept* provided previously, the use of a concept includes means of expression
and carries with it the attributes of the concept. Consequently, *use* is a
relevant focus in efforts to define the concept.

As the concept takes on a particular use, and understanding of this use
is passed on through education and socialization, the concept is applied in
a succession of new situations. Through application of the concept, its range
or scope becomes clear, along with situations that are effectively characterized using the concept. Consequently, application reveals not only the
strengths of the concept but its limitations. Based on this knowledge of the
abilities provided by the concept, directions for further development are
generated. Certain aspects of the concept undoubtedly gain significance

because of needs that exist at the time, thus stimulating the work necessary to develop, use, apply, and continually reevaluate and refine the concept.

IMPLICATIONS FOR CONCEPT DEVELOPMENT

This philosophical foundation has several significant implications for methods of concept development. The emphasis on conceptual change points to the idea that concept development must be an ongoing process, with no realistic end point, except that work on a particular concept may decrease as the concept loses significance. As phenomena, needs, and goals change, concepts must be continually refined, through whatever means are appropriate, and variations introduced to achieve a clearer and more useful repertoire. Attempts to delineate clear boundaries, to distinguish a concept from its context, or to view it apart from a network of related concepts, as often done with concept analysis, are not consistent with this view.

The emphasis on context calls attention to an important concern in the selection of settings and samples for concept development. As noted previously, the relevant context may be disciplinary, social, cultural, or theoretical. For example, inquiry into the concept of health requires the researcher to acknowledge that health may be conceptualized quite differently relative to the group membership of the person who uses the concept. Similarly, time must be considered as a factor in sample selection as historical variations are common as well.

Methods of Evolutionary Concept Analysis

The methods of concept analysis play a particularly important role in this cycle of concept development. As a result of conventional use, over time a concept may become ambiguous or vague. Some concepts may seem to be in conflict, and persons who use the concepts may not be able to describe the attributes of the concept or situations appropriate for their application. Concept analysis is focused on the *use* phase of development and is oriented toward clarification of the concept, its attributes, and its current use. Through analysis, the researcher can identify a current consensus or "state of the art" regarding the concept, which provides a foundation for further development. The focus here is on identification, an inductive approach to analysis, as the researcher seeks to identify what is common in the use of the concept, not to impose any strict criteria or expectations on the analysis.

The actual procedure of concept analysis consistent with this philosophical approach resembles the approach presented by Wilson (1963) and popularized in nursing by Walker and Avant (1983, 1988) and Chinn and Jacobs (1987; Chinn & Kramer, 1991). Nevertheless, there are important, although perhaps subtle, differences including the emphasis on an inductive inquiry and efforts to enhance the rigor of the analysis. Additional considerations arise because of the emphasis on time and context in the philosophical foundation of this approach. Because concept analysis typically is conducted using existing literature as the sample, this focus of analysis will be emphasized in this discussion.

This evolutionary method of concept analysis involves the following primary activities:

1. Identify the concept of interest and associated expressions.
2. Identify and select an appropriate realm (setting and sample) for data collection.
3. Collect data regarding the attributes of the concept, along with surrogate terms, references, antecedents, and consequences.
4. Identify concepts related to the concept of interest.
5. Analyze data regarding the above characteristics of the concept.
6. Conduct interdisciplinary or temporal comparisons, or both, if desired.
7. Identify a model case of the concept, if appropriate.
8. Identify hypotheses and implications for further development.

Many of these activities are carried out simultaneously throughout the investigation. Consequently, they represent tasks to be accomplished rather than specific steps in the process. To facilitate discussion, these activities will be described as if they are distinct.

IDENTIFYING THE CONCEPT OF INTEREST

Although this process of concept analysis is iterative, the first activity always is to identify the concept of interest and an appropriate expression. One of the most common ways of expressing a concept is through written or spoken language. Consequently, the major focus at the beginning of the study is to determine the concept of interest and appropriate terminology to guide the analysis. This is a crucial step in concept analysis, and not always as simple a task as it may seem. For example, a researcher interested in concepts applicable to a human response to a major life change may be confronted with an array of confusing concepts from which to choose, including depression, denial, sorrow, grief, and hopelessness. In a more positive view, concepts such as optimism, acceptance, coping, adaptation, accommodation, or hope might be appropriate. The selection process often is complicated by the fact that the same concept may be expressed using different terminology. Terms such as *adaptation, accommodation,* and *coping,* for example, often are used interchangeably (hence, they are surrogate terms) to express the same or, at least, a highly similar idea. Familiarity with the literature at this phase of the analysis is essential as it enables the researcher to select the concept and terminology appropriate to focus the study.

At this point in the process the researcher also must be clear about the particular direction to take with the analysis. According to this view, concept analysis always is oriented toward definition and subsequent clarification of the selected concept. Nevertheless, there are several secondary outcomes associated with clarification in general that may be of interest to the researcher and that are easily accomplished through this analysis procedure. For example, the researcher may desire to explore changes that have occurred in the concept over time or areas of agreement and disagreement across disciplines. In an exploration of the concept of health policy, I (1989b, 1989c) pursued both of these interests, examining the literature from four disciplines. This procedure revealed unique aspects of the concept of health policy as it was viewed within different fields of study and, consequently, provided useful insight into the particular perspective on health policy within each group.

In some instances, the goal might be to expand the repertoire of concepts available to characterize situations encountered in nursing practice or research. Westra and Rodgers (1991) analyzed the concept of integration for its applicability in nursing situations. Through her professional contact with chronically ill older adults in their homes, Westra had become aware of the lack of concepts applicable to these individuals as they responded to the many changes in their lives. Concepts such as coping, accommodation, or adaptation, commonly applied in such situations, did not capture effectively the interactive nature of these older adults in their relationships with their personal, physical, and social environments. Rather than merely coping with or adjusting to changes, they were much more involved in actually shaping and directing their lives, taking into account the new situations, abilities, and limitations they encountered. Mutual change, on the part of both the person and other aspects of the environment, was a prominent feature of this process.

Westra had seen references to "integration" in some of the existing literature, although it was not found in regard to the types of situations with which she was concerned. Wondering if this might be a useful way to characterize the experiences of these older adults, she pursued an analysis of the concept. As a result, we found that this concept could indeed be useful in nursing, providing an effective way of characterizing a particular human response and offering guidelines for evaluating the outcomes of nursing care (Westra & Rodgers, 1991).

CHOOSING THE SETTING AND SAMPLE

The varied goals of the evolutionary concept analysis procedure have a strong influence on selection of the setting and a sample for data collection. In a literature-based analysis the setting refers to the time period to be examined and the disciplines or types of literature to be included. As with any research, decisions related to these aspects are made based on the initial questions asked by the researcher and the desired outcomes. The ultimate goal is to generate a rigorous design consistent with the purpose of the study.

Decisions regarding which disciplines to include can be made based on familiarity with the literature and awareness of which fields of study have an interest in, and frequently employ, the concept of interest. In the analysis of the concept of health policy (Rodgers, 1989b), this concept was found to be of great interest in the fields of nursing, medicine, health care administration, and the policy sciences. Consequently, the sample was selected from the population of literature published in these domains. Similarly, in exploring the concept of integration, Westra and I (1991) drew the sample from the disciplines of education, psychology, sociology, and allied health literature for the same reasons noted above. Nursing literature also was included in this study because of our interest in the concept as it appeared in our own discipline.

For many concepts, particularly those commonly used in nursing and health care, it may be important to include the popular literature as well. Many people gain a considerable amount of information regarding health and health care through the popular media. Undoubtedly, these sources shape their individual concepts. Analysis of a concept that includes this type of literature may be beneficial in bridging the gap between the perspectives of providers and those who are the recipients of care.

When the specific domains of literature to be included in the study have been identified, the next activity involves selection of the sample to be used in the research. In studies of concepts it is not uncommon for researchers to describe their samples—if any methodological description is provided—as comprised of the literature that was either available, relevant, or pertinent to the investigation or, in some cases, to describe the sample as consisting simply of "existing literature" concerning the concept (Boyd, 1985; Brubaker, 1983; Evans, 1979; Forsyth, 1980; Matteson & Hawkins, 1990; Meize-Grochowski, 1984; Rew, 1986; Simmons, 1989; Smith, 1981). Such samples raise questions about the rigor of the design and the appropriateness of the findings. The use of literature samples offers a strong advantage to the researcher, unavailable in many types of research, in that it is possible to identify the total (indexed) population of literature through computerized data bases and printed indexes. Literature can be identified by categorical listing (i.e., major headings), by title, abstract, or key-word searches, or by a combination of these search procedures. Consequently, a more stringent sampling design may be used in the study to increase the likelihood of a credible sample.

While it is not possible to truly identify the entire population of literature using these means, it is possible to identify the total population of literature indexed. Samples drawn from this population represent a significant improvement over completely accidental or convenience samples. Furthermore, these data sources are particularly relevant for sample selection in concept analysis because of their role in institutionalizing concepts within disciplines. For example, a person in the field of education who is interested in the concept of integration is likely to consult a literature index or data base in the discipline as an early step in acquiring knowledge related to this concept. Consequently, these data bases not only contain references to literature appropriate to the concept of interest but also may work to institutionalize the use of a concept within a discipline.

Using the indexes and computer data bases to identify the total indexed population of literature, standard means of probability sampling can be used to select the sample for use in the investigation. In early studies, where my ultimate goal was to combine data from multiple disciplines to arrive at a consensus on the concept of interest, I combined the population lists and used stratified systematic sampling with a random starting point to select the actual literature items to be used in the analysis. This procedure provided a proportionate sampling from each discipline and from each year included in the design.

While this procedure has been effective, I now advocate that each discipline be treated as a separate population to facilitate more rigorous interdisciplinary comparisons for the concept of interest. A random number table or computer-generated random numbers are used to select an appropriate sample from each discipline. Like systematic sampling, this procedure requires the researcher to number each item on the list of literature, and then to select the desired number of items to represent each discipline. Generally, at least 30 items from each discipline, or 20 percent of the total population, whichever is greater, is needed, as experience has shown that this volume of literature provides an adequate basis for identifying a consensus within the discipline and for substantiating the conclusions of the researcher.

Several concerns typically emerge using this sampling design. First, there may be considerable overlap among disciplines in the literature indexed. The *Index Medicus,* for example, includes references to numerous publications that are considered representative of the nursing literature. Computerized data bases provide the capacity to delete such listings from one data base when desired, while still enabling them to appear in the appropriate population. Such overlap can also be deleted manually by the researcher's simply reviewing the printed list and eliminating or cross-referencing items that are commonly associated with another discipline (Rodgers, 1989c). Since health care is a highly interdisciplinary field, the researcher may need to make decisions regarding the treatment of journals that reflect an interdisciplinary focus. There is no rule for handling such literature, other than that the researcher have a defensible rationale and be consistent in whatever decisions are made. As interdisciplinary journals proliferate, it may be appropriate to include articles from such sources in their own stratum or, if desired, to classify the article according to the discipline of the author.

Another concern with this type of sampling procedure is related to the volume of literature that may be identified. In the study of the concept of health policy (Rodgers, 1989b, 1989c), one intent was to identify the emergence of the concept and to examine change over time. Consequently, the population included literature that spanned a 13-year period, which predated the origin of the concept and numbered 4,343 articles and 210 book reviews. This resulted in a rather cumbersome, time-consuming, and somewhat costly basis for sample selection. However, even this number of items in the total population was manageable for use in sample selection.

This particular investigation (Rodgers, 1989b, 1989c) was conducted to some extent to substantiate the view of concepts associated with this evolutionary approach; other researchers are not likely to find such a large scale analysis necessary. However, large volumes of literature are identified in many analyses, although the population and subsequent sample can be reduced to a manageable size by constricting the time frame, choice of disciplines, or choice of literature sources. Conversely, problems associated with an inadequate sample size for some concepts occasionally arise. These difficulties are overcome by expanding the scope of the study or by including other search procedures. For example, a search accomplished initially based on title alone can be expanded to include abstract and key-word searches to enlarge the population from which the sample will be selected.

There also may be some concerns related to actual indexing procedures. References sometimes are encountered that seem inappropriate to the guidelines used in the search, especially when the search is conducted using major headings. Selecting a sample of adequate size can compensate for such variances in the literature indexed. Similarly, there is the possibility that important works will be missed if the literature search is limited to computerized data bases or printed indexes alone. If the researcher feels it is appropriate, based on experience or knowledge concerning the concept of interest, works considered to be "landmark" or "classic," and special searches to identify books, book reviews, dissertations, or theses may be included (Rodgers, 1989b, 1989c). A panel of experts may be solicited as well to provide their recommendations regarding essential works on a topic (Galante, 1990; Rodgers, 1989c). The most important consideration at this stage of the investigation is to ensure a sample that is rigorously selected, with a strong rationale for all decisions, as a means to obtain effective representation of the literature and to diminish researcher bias in the study.

COLLECTING AND MANAGING THE DATA

In the evolutionary method of concept analysis the emphasis is on an inductive, discovery approach focused on identification of the relevant aspects of the concept. Consequently, the actual analysis focuses on the collection and analysis of raw data and not on the construction of "cases," as is advocated in some approaches (Walker & Avant, 1988; Wilson, 1963). The specific data collected, however, resemble that collected in other approaches to concept analysis, with minor variations. Specifically, the researcher reviews the literature to identify data relevant to the attributes, antecedents, consequences, surrogate terms, and related concepts, along with the references of the concept.

The attributes of the concept represent the primary accomplishment of concept analysis. The attributes of the concept constitute a *real* definition, as opposed to a nominal or dictionary definition that merely substitutes one synonymous expression for another (Rodgers, 1989c). It is this cluster of attributes that makes it possible to identify situations that fall under the concept, or, in other words, those that can be characterized appropriately using the concept of interest.

The researcher often has to work diligently to identify data relevant to the attributes of the concept. Actual definitions provide helpful, important data regarding the attributes, but authors rarely provide such definitions in their writing. Consequently, the researcher must look for all statements that provide a clue to how the author defines the concept. In the search for these data, it may be helpful for the researcher to keep in mind the question, What are the characteristics of (the concept)? In actual practice, the question often comes up in a more colloquial form, What is this 'thing' the writer is discussing? Any statements that provide insight into the answer to these questions constitute data relevant to the attributes.

The antecedents and consequences of the concept refer to situations, events, or phenomena that precede and follow, respectively, an example of the concept. Relevant questions to ask during this phase of data collection include, What happens before . . . ," and What happens after . . . , or as a result of (the concept)? The references indicate actual situations to which the concept is being applied. All of these outcomes of the analysis help to identify the scope of the concept to enhance its clarity and effective application.

Surrogate terms and related concepts constitute the remaining data to be collected. Surrogate terms are means of expressing the concept other than the word or expression selected by the researcher to focus the study. These terms are readily identified during data collection through the interchange of terminology. Nevertheless, the researcher must be careful to distinguish between surrogate terms and related concepts, which are concepts that bear some relationship to the concept of interest but do not seem to share the same set of attributes. In collecting these types of data it may be helpful for the researcher to keep in mind whether the author is merely using a different word for the same idea or is referring to something different altogether. The notion of surrogate terms is derived from the position that there may be multiple ways of expressing the same concept. Related concepts reflect the philosophical assumption that every single concept exists as a part of a network of related concepts that provide a background and help to impart significance to the concept of interest. Identifying these related concepts adds a contextual basis to the concept of interest.

In some approaches to concept analysis, there is an attempt to capture this idea of interconnection through the development of "related cases" (Walker & Avant, 1988; Wilson, 1963). Related cases pose some significant limitations however. First, they are constructed by the researcher, thereby providing a considerable opportunity for the introduction of bias. Most important, however, related cases are limited to a focus on application of the specific concept of interest, or situations that demonstrate perhaps some, but not all, of the attributes of the concept being analyzed. While this is an important contribution to clarifying the use of the concept of interest, it does not provide any insight into what *other* concepts might be relevant in similar situations. For example, emphasis on only related cases in the analysis of the concept of hope (Zorn, 1988) would not have revealed that optimism, faith, and so forth, are significant *concepts* to consider in viewing this human response and its potential variations. Consistent with the philosophical basis for this evolutionary perspective, the identification of related concepts is an important contribution to concept clarification overall. Significantly, this outcome can provide a useful direction to clarify additional concepts, thus adding to knowledge relevant to a broad area of concern. The work of Haase and others (see chapter 10) demonstrates further the value of identifying and clarifying related concepts.

As with any research, data management is an important concern in concept analysis, and one that is subject to numerous variations. Undoubtedly, every researcher will develop an individual style for collecting, organizing, and managing the data. In developing individual procedures, however, it is important to keep in mind both the purpose of the investigation and the analytic techniques that will be used in the study. Specifically, in recording relevant data, it is helpful to note verbatim passages in quotation marks and to note the source and page number for future reference.

The procedure that I use consists first of gathering together items selected to be included in the sample. As the literature is obtained, each item is assigned an identification number to indicate the discipline and the number of the item. Disciplines are noted using letters of the alphabet followed by the number of the item, which is the number assigned to the article on the population list. Using this identification system provides an easy means of noting a source when collecting data, helps to differentiate among the various disciplines addressed in the study, and also provides a simple cross-referencing system between each item and the original population list.

Data collection begins by reading each item at least one time to identify the general tone of the work and to gain a sense of the writer's use of the concept. This step also helps the researcher become immersed in the work, which I have found facilitates identification of data relevant to the analysis. For actual data collection I use separate sheets of paper to record data relevant to each of the major categories: attributes, antecedents, consequences, references, surrogate terms, and related concepts. Each coding sheet is identified as to both category of data and the discipline from which the data were generated. At the conclusion of data collection the data already will be organized by category to conduct analyses relevant to each significant aspect of the concept and to conduct separate analyses for each discipline to facilitate subsequent comparison.

One other type of data that is collected throughout the analysis consists of notes or records maintained by the investigator. As with any qualitative study, the researcher needs to keep track of all methodological decisions made throughout the investigation and to keep records of thoughts and perceptions as data collection and analysis proceed. Recording these impressions assists the researcher in grouping and labeling the major themes that emerge relative to each category of data and in keeping track of thoughts regarding other aspects of the analysis. Such records also provide a basis for an audit, enabling the researcher to retrace the steps of the inquiry as a means to substantiate neutrality and credibility in the investigation (Lincoln & Guba, 1985).

ANALYZING THE DATA

Although data collection and literature retrieval frequently occur simultaneously, I have found it most effective to delay the final, formal analysis until near the end of data collection. This procedure is contrary to that of most qualitative research. Nevertheless, in a typical field study, concurrent analysis is necessary to provide direction for the next step in the investigation, particularly in regard to the questions to ask and appropriate sources of data. Since there is not this same element of an emergent design in concept analysis, formal analyses may be conducted at or near the conclusion of data collection.

Undoubtedly, the researcher will have numerous thoughts and insights regarding the concept as data collection progresses, and these may be recorded appropriately in the researcher's journal. Yet, delaying formal analysis is helpful in avoiding premature closure, or jumping to conclusions, and the difficulty in seeing beyond the early impressions that may result. There are few occurrences more detrimental in concept analysis than the researcher getting stuck on a particular idea and, consequently, being unable to allow the characteristics of the concept to emerge from the data. Perhaps this avoidance of premature closure and preconceived notions—seeing what the researcher thinks the concept *should* be—presents the greatest challenge in concept analysis. It is not uncommon for investigators to select concepts that are of great interest to them, and that they would like to be able to present in a specific way after the analysis. In other words, the researcher wants the analysis to validate their pre-existing views on the concept. Since the researcher may not be totally aware of this tendency, additional measures are warranted to decrease interference from personal bias.

Concurrent analysis also seems to lead to a premature belief that the data are "saturated" when considerable redundancy is discovered. Invariably, however, the next article or book examined provides a new insight or, at least, a suggestion of a better way to express ideas related to the concept of interest. Consequently, there are considerable benefits to delaying extensive analysis until near the conclusion of data collection.

Generally, analysis is carried out according to a standard procedure of content analysis or thematic analysis. Each category of data (attributes, antecedents, consequences, and references) is examined separately to identify major themes presented in the literature. Essentially, this phase of analysis is a process of continually organizing and reorganizing similar points in the literature until a cohesive, comprehensive, and relevant system of descriptors is generated. Related concepts and surrogate terms generally are exempt from this specific analysis procedure. These typically need no further reduction, as they are recorded in simple one or two word bits of data. Nevertheless, the researcher may find it interesting to note the frequency of their occurrence in the literature examined and to make cross-disciplinary comparisons if desired.

It is unlikely that every piece of data recorded by the investigator ultimately will be clustered under some heading in the analysis phase. Certainly, the researcher will have recorded some data that seemed relevant at the time yet that on further analysis have little significance when the data are viewed collectively. Since the intent of the analysis is to identify a consensus, failure to incorporate occasional extraneous bits of information along with predominant themes is not a cause for great concern. It is inappropriate, however, to ignore data that represent "outliers" completely, as these do reveal something about the concept. Instead, they may be addressed appropriately in a discussion of the findings or, in some cases, may indicate emerging trends or the need for additional research.

As the data are organized and appropriate "labels" are identified to describe the major aspects of the concept, analysis takes on a more theoretical focus. The researcher may examine the data for areas of agreement and disagreement across disciplines, change over time, or for insight into emerging trends concerning the concept. These findings are subtle at times, yet are worth pursuing as they provide important information regarding contextual aspects of the concept, its current status, and directions for future development.

IDENTIFYING A MODEL CASE

The model case is a common part of concept analysis (Wilson, 1963). Since the evolutionary method is viewed as inductive, the model case is *identified* rather than constructed by the investigator. The purpose of the model case is to provide an example of the concept that demonstrates clearly its attributes, antecedents, and consequences (Wilson, 1963) in a relevant context. The researcher may need to review additional literature beyond the actual sample included in the study to locate a quality example of the concept. In other situations, the researcher may pursue field observations to identify a clear example of the concept.

The model case is important in providing additional clarity regarding the concept of interest. Specifically, it enhances effective application by illustrating the use of the concept in a specific situation. However, the researcher must be cautious to avoid certain pitfalls that can be associated with the model case. Foremost, as in all research, the investigator needs to maintain neutrality as much as possible. Bias can be introduced easily at this stage by the researcher's selecting examples that represent personal interests. For example, the choice of a model case related to critical care may limit the utility of the case for audiences from other settings when the results of the analysis are disseminated. Similarly, extraneous or excessive detail in the model case may distract the reader from the concept itself. The *ideal* model case is generic or universal enough to illustrate the concept clearly and in a variety of instances. Alternatively, there is no exclusion against providing more than one model case if multiple examples are available.

A more common difficulty encountered regarding the model case is the inability to locate an appropriate example. There may be a strong desire at this point to terminate the search and simply construct a case. Nevertheless, the researcher cannot consider the inability to identify an appropriate case as a limitation of the study. Instead, it reveals important information about the developmental status of the concept. It is better not to provide a model case if one cannot be found than to construct one when it is not warranted. Otherwise, the model case may promote premature closure by giving the impression that the concept is more clear, better developed, or more useful than it really is in its current state.

INTERPRETING THE RESULTS

The philosophical basis for this approach to analysis has a strong influence on the interpretation of the results. As noted previously, concept analysis is viewed here as an inductive procedure, as a means of identifying a consensus or the "state of the art" of the concept, and thus provides an important foundation for further research. The results of analysis, therefore, do not provide *the* definitive answer to questions concerning what the concept *is*. Instead, they may be viewed as a powerful heuristic, promoting and giving direction to additional inquiry. Interpretation thus proceeds along two lines: shedding insight on the current status of the concept and generating implications for inquiry based on this status and identified gaps in knowledge.

Interpretation of data regarding the current status of the concept can be pursued in many ways dependent upon the interests of the researcher. I have found cross-disciplinary comparisons to be particularly useful and enlightening in many concept analyses. In the study of the concept of health policy (Rodgers, 1989b, 1989c), a comparison of the concept across the four disciplines revealed potentially beneficial information about the perspectives of the individual disciplines. Nurse authors, for example, frequently addressed health policy in reference to health care personnel, a focus that was conspicuously absent in the literature of medicine. Identifying these differences may lead to a greater understanding of the perspectives of nurses and other professionals, recognition that not only enhances understanding across disciplines but may contribute to improved collaboration as well.

Interdisciplinary comparisons also may be useful in situations where a concept in nursing is considered to have been "borrowed" from another discipline. [The reader is referred to the large volume of nursing theory literature beginning in the late 1960s that dealt with the notion of "borrowed" versus "unique" knowledge in nursing. For example, see Johnson (1968) for historical background on this topic.] Although I do not subscribe to arguments regarding "borrowed" versus "unique" knowledge in nursing, in some situations there may be legitimate concerns about changes in perspective or the translation of the concept across contexts.

Comparisons can be conducted with regard to time as well as disciplinary contexts. Again, using health policy as an example, considerable change was noted over the 13 years of literature included in the study (Rodgers, 1989b, 1989c). Since health policy was found to be a relatively new concept, it was possible to trace its development from the superordinate concepts of public policy and social policy. In the early and mid-1970s the term *health policy* was used only rarely in the literature. The ultimate emergence of a distinct concept, along with increasing frequency in the use of this term, reflect the significance attached to this area of interest as it became a unique focus of inquiry and concern. Insight into current and emerging trends concerning the concept were gained by following the evolution of the concept over time.

IDENTIFYING IMPLICATIONS

Identification of directions for further inquiry is another important contribution of concept analysis. In fact, this heuristic function may be one of the most significant outcomes of this approach to analysis. The importance of this aspect is evident particularly in view of the philosophical foundation for this approach, which places emphasis on concept analysis as a basis for further inquiry and concept development, rather than as an end point itself.

Results of analysis of the concept of integration provide an example of the heuristic nature of this procedure (Westra & Rodgers, 1991). In this analysis, the four attributes of the concept were identified as process, combination, interaction, and unity. In other words, the concept of integration is characterized primarily as a process of combination in which two or more elements interact and form a new, unified entity (Westra & Rodgers, 1991).

Based on this analysis, a number of questions and areas for further research were identified. Field studies constitute one important area for research to evaluate the utility of the concept in actual nursing situations or to gather data for further clarification of the concept. This focus is consistent with the concept development procedure presented by Schwartz-Barcott and Kim (1986; see chapter 8), which combines a literature-based analysis with a fieldwork phase. For the concept of integration, fieldwork might be conducted to determine the incidence of integration and its presence or applicability in actual nursing situations. Similarly, research could be designed to address questions concerning how people perceive their experiences in *integrating* various aspects of their lives, such as the combination of a previous sense of self with an altered self following some life change. Additional questions might be focused on newly acquired roles and relationships and the integration of a person with an altered functional status within an able society.

In addition to the many possibilities for productive fieldwork suggested by this analysis, further research may be facilitated by hypotheses derived from the analysis. Hypotheses regarding a variety of factors associated with integration may be tested using experimental or quasi-experimental designs. Such research could include the development and testing of nursing interventions designed to promote integration. Similarly, for integration, criteria can be identified to assess the presence of integration as an outcome of nursing care or as a means for instrument development (Westra & Rodgers, 1991).

Certainly, such research might be conducted without a prior analysis of the concept. Nevertheless, an initial analysis can enhance research by providing a solid conceptual foundation for further study. As a part of this process, it also provides a mechanism for systematic review of a large volume of literature. Finally, concept analysis can serve as a strong basis for substantiating the need for a particular study, particularly in regard to hypotheses and significant gaps in knowledge that are identified as a result of the analysis.

Conclusion

Concept analysis has an important role in the development of the knowledge base of nursing. However, there are numerous approaches to analysis, each with its own philosophical foundation. A philosophical foundation is implicit in many instances, yet has a profound effect on the conduct of the analysis and the interpretation and utilization of results.

The evolutionary approach to analysis is based on current philosophical thought regarding concepts and their role in knowledge development (Ryle,

1971; Toulmin, 1972; Wittgenstein, 1953/1968). This foundation emphasizes the dynamic nature of concepts, changing with both time and context. In addition, it is consistent with the idea that vast interrelationships exist among phenomena and among the concepts that are associated with them. In general, this approach represents the philosophical rejection of essentialism and absolutism, which were prevalent in regard to concepts and knowledge during the first half of the twentieth century. Instead, concepts are considered to change, grow, and develop (and need to be developed) in an evolutionary manner to enhance and maintain clarity and utility in the discipline.

This philosophical basis, with all the attendant assumptions about conceptual change and the role of context, has significant implications for the actual method of concept analysis. Emphasis is placed especially on the conduct of a rigorous and systematic study. Specific considerations have been noted in regard to sample selection or literature review, an aspect of concept analysis that has not received adequate attention in the majority of discussions. Interpretation of the results of analysis is guided by this foundation as well, revealing the heuristic value of concept analysis.

At present, this evolutionary view of concept analysis offers several advantages for the researcher doing the analysis, and provides a viable alternative to existing procedures. It has been used successfully with literature-based analyses of concepts as diverse as health policy (Rodgers, 1989b, 1989c); hope (Zorn, 1988); grief (Rodgers & Cowles, 1991; see chapter 7); integration (Westra & Rodgers, 1991); family (Cook, 1990); behavior change (Ryan, 1990); strategic management (Galante, 1990); and hardiness (Nesbitt, 1992); to name a few. I have encouraged, as well, analyses based on interview data rather than the usual literature approach. Currently, Cowles (personal communication, July 1, 1991) is employing this approach using focus groups comprised of members of different cultures for further exploration of the concept of grief. This technique promises to be particularly valuable in clarification of cultural differences concerning the concept of interest.

There is a need for a variety of approaches to concept development. Additional investigations using this approach with a variety of types of concepts will be helpful in further refining this method and demonstrating the scope of its applicability. Ideally, this will contribute to further progress in concept development in nursing.

REFERENCES

Barsalou, L. W., & Medin, D. L. (1986). Concepts: Static definitions or context-dependent representations? *Cahiers de Psychologie Cognitive, 6,* 187–202.
Boyd, C. (1985). Toward an understanding of mother-daughter identification using concept analysis. *Advances in Nursing Science, 7*(3), 78–86.

Brubaker, B. H. (1983). Health promotion: A linguistic analysis. *Advances in Nursing Science,* 5(3), 1–14.

Chinn, P. L., & Jacobs, M. K. (1987). *Theory and nursing: A systematic approach.* St. Louis: Mosby.

Chinn, P. L., & Kramer, M. (1991). *Theory and nursing: A systematic approach* (3rd ed). St. Louis: Mosby.

Cook, A. (1990). *The concept of family.* Unpublished manuscript.

Evans, S. K. (1979). Descriptive criteria for the concept of depleted health potential. *Advances in Nursing Science, 1*(3), 67–74.

Fehr, B. (1988). Prototype analysis of the concepts of love and commitment. *Journal of Personality and Social Psychology, 55,* 557–579.

Forsyth, G. L. (1980). Analysis of the concept of empathy: Illustration of one approach. *Advances in Nursing Science, 2*(2), 33–42.

Galante, C. (1990). *Strategic management in nursing: A concept analysis.* Unpublished doctoral dissertation, George Mason University, Fairfax, Virginia.

Johnson, D. E. (1968). Theory in nursing: Borrowed or unique? *Nursing Research, 17,* 206–209.

Lincoln, Y. S., & Guba, E. (1985). *Naturalistic inquiry.* Beverly Hills: Sage.

Matteson, P., & Hawkins, J. W. (1990). Concept analysis of decision-making. *Nursing Forum, 25*(2), 4–10.

McCloskey, M. E., & Glucksberg, S. (1978). Natural categories: Well defined or fuzzy sets? *Memory & Cognition, 6,* 462–472.

Meize-Grochowski, R. (1984). An analysis of the concept of trust. *Journal of Advanced Nursing, 9,* 563–572.

Nesbitt, B. (1992). *Analysis of the concept of hardiness.* Unpublished manuscript.

Price, H. H. (1953). *Thinking and experience.* London: Hutchinson House.

Rew, L. (1986). Intuition: Concept analysis of a group phenomenon. *Advances in Nursing Science, 8*(2), 21–28.

Rodgers, B. L. (1989a). Concepts, analysis, and the development of nursing knowledge: The evolutionary cycle. *Journal of Advanced Nursing, 14,* 330–335.

Rodgers, B. L. (1989b). Exploring health policy as a concept. *Western Journal of Nursing Research, 11,* 694–702.

Rodgers, B. L. (1989c). The use and applications of concepts in nursing: The case of health policy (Doctoral dissertation, University of Virginia, 1987). *Dissertation Abstracts International, 49–11B,* 4756.

Rodgers, B. L., & Cowles, K. V. (1991). The concept of grief: An analysis of classical and contemporary thought. *Death Studies, 15,* 443–458.

Ryan, P. (1990). *The concept of behavior change.* Unpublished manuscript.

Ryle, G. (1971). *Collected papers* (Vols. 1–2). London: Hutchinson House.

Schwartz-Barcott, D., & Kim, H. S. (1986). A hybrid model for concept development. In P. L. Chinn (Ed.). *Nursing Research Methodology: Issues and Implementation* (pp. 91–101). Rockville, Md: Aspen.

Simmons, S. J. (1989). Health: A concept analysis. *International Journal of Nursing Studies, 26,* 155–161.

Smith, J. A. (1981). The idea of health: A philosophical inquiry. *Advances in Nursing Science, 3*(3), 43–50.

Smith, E. E., & Medin, D. L. (1981). *Categories and concepts.* Cambridge, Mass: Harvard University.

Toulmin, S. (1972). *Human understanding.* Princeton, NJ: Princeton University.

Walker, L. O., & Avant, K. C. (1983). *Strategies for theory construction in nursing.* Norwalk, Conn: Appleton-Century-Crofts.

Walker, L. O., & Avant, K. C. (1988). *Strategies for theory construction in nursing* (2nd ed.). Norwalk, Conn: Appleton & Lange.

Westra, B. L., & Rodgers, B. L. (1991). Integration: A concept for evaluating outcomes of nursing care. *Journal of Professional Nursing, 7,* 277–282.

Wilson, J. (1963). *Thinking with concepts.* London: Cambridge University Press.

Wittgenstein, L. (1968). *Philosophical investigations* (3rd ed.; G. E. M. Anscombe, Trans.). Chicago: University of Chicago Press. (Original work published 1953)

Zorn, C. (1988). *The concept of hope.* Unpublished manuscript.

Chapter 7

The Concept of Grief: An Evolutionary Perspective

KATHLEEN V. COWLES AND BETH L. RODGERS

*T*he concept of grief has been of interest to both practitioners and researchers from a wide variety of disciplines for many years. It has been compared to and contrasted with depression, it has been equated with "melancholia" (Freud, 1917/1957), and it has been variously defined as an adaptational response (Bowlby, 1973), as an acute crisis or a series of crises (Caplan, 1974; Lindemann, 1944), as an illness (Engel, 1961; Volkan, 1970), as a syndrome (Lindemann, 1944; Parkes, 1972), and as a human response (Kim, McFarland, & McLane, 1989). Psychologists, psychiatrists, general medical practitioners, nurses, sociologists, veterinarians, educators, and theologians have all written about grief and the importance of understanding this universal experience. Despite the agreement across disciplines regarding the significance of the phenomenon of grief and despite the proliferation of multidisciplinary professional literature describing instances of its occurrence, there continues to be evidence in the literature that the concept of grief is vague and ambiguous and that, in fact, there is little agreement either within or between disciplines on a conceptual definition of grief.

In 1989 we completed a concept analysis of grief that was designed to systematically identify a definition of the concept as it had been used in the literature of nursing and medicine (Cowles & Rodgers, 1991). In addition to identifying a definition of grief, we traced the historical and contextual development of the concept and determined the areas of agreement and disagreement concerning grief as it had been conceptualized in the literature of these two disciplines.

The analysis revealed that the concept of grief covered a wide range of responses and experiences. The authors seldom provided an actual definition of *grief;* instead, they typically discussed grief in relation to a multitude of common, observable, and reported symptoms. In addition, many authors

93

used a variety of terms other than *grief* to express their individual concepts and often used qualifiers to indicate subtle variations in the concept.

Despite the wide variety of approaches to the discussion of grief in both the medical and nursing literature, it was possible to identify the predominant attributes of the concept. The identification of these attributes resulted in the definition of grief as a *dynamic, pervasive, highly individualized process with a strong normative component* (Rodgers & Cowles, 1991). While this conceptualization offered a significant contribution to the development of a knowledge base concerning grief in medicine and nursing, we decided that further study and clarification was warranted, particularly in light of the numerous disciplinary references to sociology and psychology and to specific authors from these disciplines throughout the literature of nursing and medicine. Therefore, a second phase of the analysis was focused on the literature of sociology and psychology and was completed in 1990. The remainder of this chapter is devoted to a discussion of the method of concept analysis used in these investigations, the interdisciplinary comparison of the findings, and the merged results of these studies.

Concept Analysis Method

Rodgers (1987, 1989a, 1989b) advocated a method of concept analysis that is an inductive, descriptive means of inquiry used to clarify the current status of a concept by identifying a consensus, to examine the historical or evolutionary background of the concept, and to determine areas of agreement and disagreement in the use of the concept among diverse disciplines. We strictly adhered to this method throughout both phases of the study.

SAMPLE SELECTION

The samples for both phases were selected from English language literature published in the respective fields of medicine, nursing, psychology, and sociology during the years 1985 through 1988. Initially the population of indexed literature was identified through a manual search of the *Index Medicus* and the *International Nursing Index,* as these indexes represented important reference sources for these two disciplines. Medicine and nursing constituted the focus of the first phase of the study because of our primary interest in conceptualizations of grief in these two fields of study. The search was accomplished by identifying all literature indexed under the subject headings *grief* and *bereavement,* as these two terms frequently are used interchangeably in the literature in this topic area. Cross-referencing between indexes was eliminated through a manual review of the total population identified in each field. A computer search could have been used to accomplish this task. However, a computer search based on major headings would have produced a list identical to that published in the indexes. Consequently, a manual search was considerably less costly to use in this investigation. We also knew that there would be a sizable volume of literature indexed under the major headings of *grief* and *bereavement;* thus there was no need to expand the search by using key words, an abstract search, or other means of literature retrieval.

This initial search uncovered 242 items in the *Index Medicus* and 159 in the nursing literature. For ease of sample selection and to maintain a master list of the literature, the relevant pages from each index were photocopied and each discipline was assigned a letter for differentiation of the populations. Each data base was treated as separate, and the articles listed were numbered sequentially in each population. A sample was selected from each discipline (nursing, n = 30; medicine, n = 44) using computer-generated random numbers. In determining the sample size, the investigators first selected 30 as the target number of items to be selected from the smaller data base of nursing. Experience had shown that 30 items was the minimum needed to facilitate a credible analysis (Rodgers, 1987, 1989a, 1989b). The investigators recognized that more articles could be added if needed to identify a consensus. Since this sample size constituted approximately 18 percent of the literature identified in nursing, a corresponding sample of 18 percent of the literature indexed in medicine was selected. This same procedure was used later in selecting the samples from sociology and psychology using the *Social Sciences Index* (N = 150, n = 30, 20 percent) and *Psych Abstracts* (N = 547, n = 109, 20 percent).

A purposive sample of works considered to be landmark or classic was included as well. For this study, this sample was identified through a review of the citations in the articles selected from each discipline. The most frequently cited references were selected to comprise this sample of classics. This sample included works by Bowlby (1980), Engel (1964), Lindemann (1944), and Parkes (1972, 1975), along with a chapter on conceptualizations of grief drawn from psychology, psychoanalysis, pastoral care, and medicine (Switzer, 1970). It may be of interest to note that works by Kubler-Ross (1969) were not included in this selection of classics. Although these works were cited frequently in the nursing literature on grief, they did not appear in the reference lists for articles selected from other disciplines. In addition, Kubler-Ross focused her work on death and dying, and not on a discussion of grief or bereavement.

LITERATURE RETRIEVAL AND DATA COLLECTION

After the sample was selected, we obtained the literature through local libraries and interlibrary loan services. Each item was read initially to identify the general tone and theme of the work. This step helped focus our attention on the task of data collection, to become immersed in the literature, and to become sensitized to the authors' uses of the concept of grief. Phrases, themes, and, when possible, verbatim passages were recorded onto coding sheets developed to organize the data. For example, a coding form with the heading "Definitions" was used to document all data relevant to the question What are the attributes of the concept of grief? Similar coding forms were used to record data relevant to other aspects of data collection as well (antecedents, consequences, references, related concepts, and surrogate terms). A separate set of coding forms was used for each discipline represented in the study. As relevant data were noted on the appropriate form, the complete item number from which the data were extracted was noted as well. Page numbers also were included, which made it possible for us to return to the original source of the data if additional clarification was needed. We reviewed each others' data collection and recording processes at intervals throughout the study to ensure a consistent approach to the inquiry and as a form of peer review (Lincoln & Guba, 1985) to diminish potential bias in the investigation.

Occasionally during data collection, the data obtained in each discipline were reviewed and reorganized as some categories began to emerge. Analysis was limited until near the end of data collection, however, to avoid premature closure regarding the relevant aspects of the concept. Instead, the minimal analysis conducted throughout the study was done primarily to promote organization of the data, which also facilitated later, formal analysis.

DATA ANALYSIS

As the actual investigation was conducted in two stages, data analysis also was carried out in two phases. Analysis first was focused on the nursing and medical literature, with the data from each discipline analyzed separately. Then the results of these analyses were combined to reveal a working definition of the concept. As noted previously, this analysis led to the second phase focused on the disciplines of sociology and psychology. Data from sociology and psychology also were reviewed separately, and then combined with the results of the first phase analysis to provide greater clarity and an expanded and more comprehensive definition of the concept. Finally, the data and findings were scrutinized to examine areas of agreement and disagreement among the four disciplines, and to examine conceptual change over time.

In this study, analysis was carried out in an inductive, thematic manner similar to content analysis. Data collected within each discipline were analyzed relevant to the major categories of information recorded. In other words, all data recorded under the heading "Definitions" for one discipline were analyzed to identify a definition (the attributes) of the concept of grief; this same procedure was followed for antecedents, consequences, references, surrogate terms, and related concepts. Data were organized and reorganized until a coherent system of categories emerged for each aspect of the concept. Word labels then were selected to provide clear descriptions of each aspect of the concept, using actual words obtained from the data when appropriate. The only exceptions to this process were the surrogate terms and related concepts. Because data under these headings typically were noted as one- or two-word expressions, rather than as general themes or phrases, there was no need for categorizing and labeling; these data were in a final form as collected on the coding sheets. However, frequency counts were used on a limited basis to describe the findings in these areas, and some analysis was conducted to clarify relationships between the concept of interest, surrogate terms, and other related concepts.

Consistent with this approach to concept analysis (Rodgers, 1987, 1989a, 1989b), the actual analysis was focused generally on identification of a consensus to reveal the "state of the art," or the current state of knowledge, concerning the concept. Consequently, some data noted on the coding sheets were not incorporated into the final category system, especially in regard to the definition or attributes of the concept. The utilization of every piece of data recorded constitutes one of the most frequent concerns or questions of persons conducting this type of inquiry. Undoubtedly, each investigator noted some information that, during the analysis, was found to shed little light on the characteristics of the concept. This occurrence is common particularly because of the guideline used in this type of analysis that if some information seems even potentially relevant, it is better to note it on the data collection sheet than to risk losing the data altogether. As commonly occurs, some of the data collected in this study ultimately were found to be irrelevant, especially as the concept became more clear through analysis.

Another common situation, which also emerged during this study, involved some small bits of data that did not fit the category system that was developed to incorporate the majority of the data. Yet, these data were too important to be discarded as irrelevant. Since the emphasis here was on consensus, the categories generally were developed to incorporate as much of the data as possible and, certainly, to capture the dominant ideology. The remaining data provided significant insights regarding the concept nonetheless. These "outliers" were found to represent the remnants of earlier ideas, ideas outside of the mainstream (e.g., frequent references in nursing to the stages of grief purportedly addressed by Kubler-Ross), or emerging trends. Focused attention on these data, such as by examining their context in the literature sources, reference citations, background of author, and relationship of these ideas to others found in the literature, helped in determining the significance of this information in reference to the current status of the concept and the cycle of concept development.

Throughout all aspects of the study, strategies relevant to qualitative research were used to enhance the credibility of the findings (Lincoln & Guba, 1985). Each investigator maintained a reflexive journal as a record of all methodological decisions and as documentation of impressions that emerged during data collection and analysis. In addition, the involvement of two researchers helped to decrease the influence of individual biases in the research. The absence of any hypotheses in the conduct of the study also enhanced neutrality in this investigation. Finally, the rigor of the study was supported through the use of a probability sample and an adequate sample size to enable convergence of the data.

Findings

The first, and perhaps most obvious, finding of this study was the tremendous variety of ways in which the concept of grief commonly was used. We had sufficient evidence prior to the study to document vagueness and ambiguity and the need for clarification and further development of the concept of grief. Yet, this investigation revealed a striking array of uses and interpretations of this concept.

Few authors provided an actual definition of *grief;* instead, grief was commonly discussed in regard to symptoms and interventions. In addition, the term *grief* frequently was interchanged with a variety of surrogate terms, most often *mourning* and *bereavement.* These terms also were defined only rarely by the authors of the literature examined. Finally, grief commonly was used in conjunction with a variety of modifiers, including *complicated, pathological,* and *dysfunctional* grief, *normal* or *typical* grief, and *anticipatory, atypical,* and *disenfranchised* grief.

ATTRIBUTES OF GRIEF

Even with this wide variety of approaches to grief, there was some consensus on the concept. Analysis of the literature in the disciplines of nursing and medicine resulted in the definition of the concept of grief as a dynamic, pervasive, highly individualized process with a strong normative component (Rodgers & Cowles, 1991). This listing of attributes—dynamic, individualized, pervasive, process, and normative—was consistent throughout the literature in sociology and psychology as well. In fact, the "labels" selected for the attributes often were found in the literature examined in the second part of this investigation. Before the second phase, we put much thought into selecting appropriate descriptors for the attributes and into choosing labels that would best capture the nature of the attribute. On examination of the sociology and psychology literature, some of the actual terms selected to describe the attributes were found, particularly the terms *pervasive* and *dynamic.* The term *process* was used in some of the literature in all four disciplines, although less frequently in nursing. *Normative* was derived on the basis of numerous authors' discussions of *normal* or *typical* grief and of acceptable or appropriate grief responses in addition to some limited reference to cultural variations in regard to grief.

Dynamic. Most discussions of grief presented this concept as representing a nonlinear, fluctuating complex of emotions, thoughts, and behaviors. Although grief commonly was regarded as having distinct phases, there were many different descriptions of the nature of these phases. Some authors (Green & Goldberg, 1986; Zisook & DeVaul, 1985) did refer to grief as characterized by certain "steps" and a linear progression. However, these authors typically relied on older references as the sources for this idea. The more current use of the concept provided evidence of an increasing conceptualization of grief as constantly changing and, thus, dynamic in nature.

Also significant in regard to this attribute was an interdisciplinary difference noted as a part of this analysis. Frequent references to the work of Kubler-Ross (1969) and her portrayal of the stages of the *dying* process, which was used as a means to understand both dying and grieving, created a skew in the nursing literature away from the more contemporary idea of grief as dynamic and nonlinear. Rarely did references to Kubler-Ross appear in the literature of medicine, and they were not found at all in discussions of grief in the literature from sociology and psychology that was examined in this study.

Process. The attribute *process* is closely related to the attribute *dynamic.* The frequent reference to grief as characterized by phases or clusters of activity in movement toward some goal revealed the process aspect of this concept. A similar major idea expressed in the literature concerned grief as "work" (Clark, 1984; Elde, 1986; Martocchio, 1985; Worden, 1985). The work of grief consisted of a variety of tasks related to reconciliation of a loss or progression to get beyond the impact and effects of the loss. There was considerable disagreement about the amount of time needed for a person to complete the work of grief. Earlier ideas presented the grief process as approximately six months to two years in duration. Nevertheless, there was an emerging, and increasing, consensus that grief is potentially without any time limit. The enduring nature of grief is particularly evident in discussions of how significant events and other reminders of a loss serve to revive aspects of grief for many years (Paterson, 1987; Zisook & DeVaul, 1985).

Individualized. Authors of the literature reviewed presented a tremendous variety of both objective and subjective experiences associated with the occurrence of grief. The specific combination of experiences was thought to differ among individuals, with the particular experiences of a person affected by numerous factors including the relationship between the grieving person and the lost being or object, the nature of the loss (e.g., traumatic, acute, predicted), and existing support systems. Other factors, such as the individual's previous experience with loss and grief, culture, and religious beliefs also were presented as having a strong effect on grief. Overall, it was clear that the concept of grief is highly individualized, and manifested in many different ways from one person to the next. Some authors did attempt to provide a list of symptoms common to all persons experiencing grief (Lesher & Bergey, 1988; Norris & Murrell, 1987), and in fact, such symptoms often were advocated as definitive in nature. This analysis, however, clearly revealed that there was little agreement on any specific set of symptoms associated with grief. The general consensus was that grief is highly individualized in nature.

Pervasive. In addition to being highly individualized, the concept of grief also was considered to be pervasive, having the potential to affect every aspect of a person's existence. Grief may manifest in ways that can be classified as psychological, social, physical, cognitive, behavioral, spiritual, and emotional or affective. This tremendous range of possible experiences and manifestations associated with grief provides evidence of the pervasive attribute of this concept. Almost any combination, magnitude, or duration of manifestations is possible as a part of the concept of grief; more often than not, multiple aspects of a grieving person's existence are affected.

Normative. Although there was a consensus that grief is highly variable, there was a tremendous tendency on the part of the authors of the literature examined to identify what constituted *normal* grief. Authors frequently used terms such as *typical, uncomplicated,* and *healthy* grief, in addition to *normal,* to differentiate an expected or acceptable response from one that might be considered *complicated, pathological,* or *atypical.* Although there was not universal agreement as to what constituted *normal* grief, there was a clear consensus that there are limits beyond which grief becomes unacceptable or inappropriate. These limits commonly were discussed as being socially or culturally ascribed. The argument was made often that an individual essentially learns how to grieve as a part of socialization and enculturation processes.

ANTECEDENTS

All the literature examined revealed that the primary antecedent, or situation preceding an instance of the concept of grief, was some form of loss. We were not surprised to find that the type of loss most frequently addressed was the death of a significant other, especially a family member. There was, however, a considerable variety of losses discussed by the authors of the works included in this study. Some of these other losses associated with grief were relatively tangible in nature, such as physical dysfunction or impairment, the loss of a pet, or the loss of some significant object. Other losses were more abstract, such as the loss of independence or control, losses associated with aging or a change in lifestyle or residence, and, less frequently noted in the literature, divorce, menopause, retirement, the loss of an idealized child (through infertility or birth defects), and loss of employment.

Some of these losses actually were described by authors in terms of *change,* such as a change in residence or employment or changes experienced in conjunction with aging. The emphasis on change in the literature was sufficient for us to consider it as another antecedent of the concept of grief. Nevertheless, further analysis revealed that change, alone, was not the antecedent; rather, it was the losses associated with change that may lead to grief. Consequently, the antecedent of loss subsumed all of the antecedents presented in the literature. By far, the antecedent most often discussed involved the death of a loved one.

CONSEQUENCES

The consequences of grief, or situations that follow an instance of the concept, were difficult to discern in this analysis. Problems with this aspect of the inquiry were related to an interesting characteristic of the literature on grief, specifically the tendency of authors to refer to specific symptoms of grief as the outcomes or consequences. For example, authors frequently indicated that grief "results" in sadness, crying, loss of concentration, and a variety of somatic disturbances. However, for purposes of this analysis, attention was focused on the more long-range outcomes of grief. These other "results" of grief are more properly considered as symptoms or manifestations. These symptoms occur while the individual is grieving. Thus, they do not answer the question concerning what happens to a person as a result of a grief experience, in other words, to someone who has made considerable movement through the grief process.

Two consequences of grief were identified: the development of a new identity and the establishment of a new reality. Typically, as a consequence of grief, a new personal and social identity emerge as the grieving individual reconceptualizes the self without the lost object (or person). Alterations in roles, activities, and routines, along with changes in social relationships, frequently occur. Ultimately, "life is never the same" (Karl, 1987, p. 645) for the person who has experienced grief, an expression that illustrates clearly the magnitude and extent of the outcome of grief in altering the person's identity and reality.

The consequences of grief were discussed most often in reference to effects on the grieving person. Nevertheless, the analysis demonstrated that a grief experience may have an effect beyond the impact on the persons actually grieving. Particularly, grief was noted by a few authors (Beckey, Price, Okerson, & Riley, 1985; Kowalski, 1985) to have an effect on health care systems and professional care providers. Interestingly, however, this position was identified only in the nursing literature. Authors occasionally pointed out that health care delivery may be changed somewhat as a result of a grief experience in a setting, and may include new interventions to assist grieving persons. Physical structures may be altered, for example, the development of privacy rooms for grieving family members on nursing units. Significantly, nurse authors also noted that health care personnel may be affected by an experience with grief either by the self or by others in the work setting, especially clients. An encounter with grief may contribute to feelings of inadequacy or helplessness, and may lead to questioning of personal beliefs, faith, and individual well-being and mortality in persons associated with a grieving individual.

RELATED CONCEPTS

As noted previously, various terms were used interchangeably to express the concept of grief. Some of these terms actually were found to express related concepts, in addition to functioning as surrogate terms for *grief.* This determination was made based on an analysis that revealed sometimes subtle differences in expressions as well as authors who provided more precise definitions of alternate terms. For example, *bereavement* was defined as "the state of having experienced the death of a significant other" (Demi & Miles, 1986, p. 105). Similarly, *mourning,* another term frequently used interchangeably with *grief,* has been used specifically to refer to the rituals and practices that serve as a public display of grief (Parkes, 1985). Bereavement and mourning thus bear a close relationship to grief, yet could be used effectively to refer to specific aspects of a grief experience. Although such terms were presented frequently as surrogates, there was a distinct difference in the attributes of each associated concept. This interchange of terms not only adds to confusion in this area, but undermines the effectiveness of these various ways of characterizing unique aspects of a grief experience.

The Evolution of Grief as a Concept

In addition to addressing common aspects of concept analysis, as well as interdisciplinary variations, we also examined changes that had occurred in the concept of grief over time. The purposive sample of landmark works utilized for this aspect of the analysis included six classic publications selected on the basis of frequency of citation as references in the contemporary literature. Analysis for this aspect of the study revealed that there has been little change in the concept of grief over time. Tremendous variation in discussions of grief was evident, and rarely was a definition of grief provided. Symptoms of grief provided the primary focus for authors of much of the classic literature, and terms were interchanged freely, both of which were apparent in contemporary writings as well.

Some subtle tendencies were noted in this aspect of the analysis, however, including a gradually expanding view of the duration and antecedents of grief. Although there was not uniform agreement among authors on the subject, there was some evidence that the time involved for resolution of grief is being viewed as less restrictive (for example, potentially limitless rather than persisting for only six months or so, after which grief may be "pathological"). Similarly, there has been a gradual increase in attention to grief in response to a variety of losses, rather than death of a significant other alone, although the primary emphasis continues to be on loss associated with death. Overall, there has been little progress in abilities to conceptualize grief clearly in development of a consensus and, particularly, in the ability to recognize or identify grief and differentiate grief from other related responses.

Implications

The lack of progress concerning the concept of grief, despite many years of inquiry, is one of the best indicators of the need for this analysis. The results of this study provide a foundation for the additional development of the concept that is needed. Particularly, these findings offer not only some of the needed clarity but serve a heuristic purpose in facilitating productive inquiry.

The definition of the concept of grief that was derived through this analysis may help providers who need to identify grief and differentiate it from related responses. One of the most significant outcomes of this analysis was the observation that grief cannot be identified on the basis of symptoms alone. Although symptomatology has been a focus in discussions of grief for many years, essentially there was no agreement on symptoms commonly or properly associated with grief. The highly variable and individualized nature of grief indicates that recognition of this response is best based on an individual's antecedent loss and the person's own description of his or her experience as *grief*. Grief is quite complex and varied such that an emphasis on symptoms alone is inadequate to enable identification of this response.

This finding obviously has implications for the development of nursing diagnoses concerning grief and related responses. Undoubtedly, determining a discrete set of defining characteristics is complicated by the myriad and highly individualized forms of grief. Furthermore, without a clear conceptualization of grief, it is difficult, and premature as well, to label or identify cases as "anticipatory" or "dysfunctional" grief. These existing diagnoses are vague and demonstrate considerable overlap, both of which limit their usefulness in clinical situations. Further research is needed before valid diagnostic statements can be developed and implemented.

Research using interviews is needed to enhance knowledge of appropriate interventions for grief. Currently, there is a sizable volume of literature that is focused on counseling and other therapeutic activities for grieving persons. Nevertheless, there is minimal agreement on the interventions that are warranted, on the timing for implementation, and, in fact, on the appropriateness of any interventions in situations of grief. Interview-based research also may be helpful in clarifying the normative aspect of grief. Cross-cultural studies particularly are needed to shed light on cultural norms and to expand the currently limited knowledge on this topic.

In spite of the significance of interview-based research in expanding understanding of grief, other aspects of this analysis generated hypotheses and other directives to promote additional forms of inquiry. The identification of loss as the primary antecedent points to the need for research regarding grief responses in association with various types of loss. Although there is some research that suggests grief may vary in relation to the acuity or prior knowledge of an impending loss, less information is available regarding specific differences in response to losses other than the death of a significant other. Losses associated with the institutionalization of a loved one, the loss of a significant object, and more abstract losses including the loss of a previous sense of self, independence, and personal functions have been studied to a much lesser extent. Since the concept of grief was found in this analysis to be highly individualized, research to uncover some of the factors that influence individual variations is needed.

The consequences of grief identified through this analysis provide direction for additional research as well. In addition to their potential use in assessing progression through the grief process, these consequences offer a reconceptualization and a basis for evaluation of grief outcomes. Previously, research on the outcomes, or consequences, of grief had been limited primarily to a focus on symptom resolution. Research to develop means that are more precise to address changes in individual identity and reality ultimately would increase understanding of the dynamic nature of progression through a grief experience.

Attention needs also to be focused on the variety of related concepts and surrogate terms identified through this analysis. The frequent interchange of terms has contributed substantially to the existing confusion and ambiguity concerning the concept of grief. Similarly, it has created difficulties in synthesizing the results of research due to vast conceptual differences in studies of grief. It is important to recognize as well that many of these terms can be used effectively to address specific and important aspects of a response to loss. Clarification of terminology and associated concepts, especially the concepts of mourning and bereavement, would be a major step in advancing knowledge of grief. In addition, there is a need for attention to related concepts that refer to various types of grief, such as pathological or complicated. Analysis of these concepts, along with empirical research focused on grief experiences, can promote differentiation of these concepts and contribute to a broader knowledge base and, certainly, more useful and relevant concepts overall.

A prior analysis of the concept is not essential in conducting research along any of these lines. Nevertheless, analysis of the concept of grief was helpful in identifying the "state of the art," so to speak, in determining aspects of the concept that particularly need refining and in providing clear directions for inquiry. Ultimately, such an analysis enables additional research to be conducted with a strong conceptual foundation and to be potentially more productive as the inquiry is focused on specific deficiencies in knowledge. The method used in this investigation particularly strengthens future research efforts through its systematic approach to sample selection and literature review, attention to the evolution of the concept, and a focus on interdisciplinary analyses and comparisons. These factors contribute to a rigorous study and a multitude of useful outcomes.

Still, the results of this analysis do not specifically answer questions about what grief *is*. Indeed, the philosophical basis for the approach used in this study rejects the idea that any one definitive answer could exist. Concepts are not timeless, acontextual entities, but reflect a changing world and continuing alterations in their use. The method used in this analysis of the concept of grief differs from other approaches by emphasizing this philosophical assumption and by focusing on the current use of the concept. This method serves to clarify the current status of the concept and thus promotes the concept's more effective use and application. Further analyses are needed to clarify the array of related concepts to expand knowledge of this broad area of interest. Equally important, however, is the need for continuing research and development of the concept of grief to maintain a concept that is clear, useful, and relevant. This analysis can be considered a starting point for additional productive inquiry.

REFERENCES

Beckey, R. D., Price, R. A., Okerson, M., & Riley, K. W. (1985). Development of a perinatal grief checklist. *Journal of Obstetric, Gynecologic and Neonatal Nursing, 14,* 194–199.

Bowlby, J. (1973). *Attachment and loss: Vol. 2. Separation, anxiety and anger.* New York: Basic Books.

Bowlby, J. (1980). *Attachment and loss: Vol. 3. Loss.* New York: Basic Books.

Caplan, G. (1974). Foreword. In I. Glick, R. Weiss, & C. Parkes (Eds.), *The first year of bereavement* (pp. vi–xi). New York: Wiley.

Clark, M. D. (1984). Healthy and unhealthy grief behaviors. *Occupational Health Nursing, 32,* 633–635.

Cowles, K. V., & Rodgers, B. L. (1991). The concept of grief: A foundation for nursing practice and research. *Research in Nursing and Health, 14,* 119–127.

Demi, A. S., & Miles, M. G. (1986). Bereavement. *Annual Review of Nursing Research, 4,* 105–123.

Elde, C. (1986). The use of multiple group therapy in support groups for grieving families. *American Journal of Hospice Care, 3*(6), 27–31.

Engel, G. L. (1961). Is grief a disease: A challenge for medical research. *Psychosomatic Medicine, 23,* 18–22.

Engel, G. L. (1964). Grief and grieving. *American Journal of Nursing, 64,* 93–98.

Freud, S. (1957). Mourning and melancholia. In J. Strachey (Ed. and Trans.), *The standard edition of the complete psychological works of Sigmund Freud* (Vol. 14, pp. 243–258). London: Hogarth. (Original work published 1917)

Green, S. A., & Goldberg, R. L. (1986). Management of acute grief. *American Family Physician, 33,* 185–190.

Karl, G. R. (1987). A new look at grief. *Journal of Advanced Nursing, 12,* 641–645.

Kim, M. J., McFarland, G. K., & McLane, A. M. (1989). *Pocket guide to nursing diagnoses* (3rd ed.). St. Louis: Mosby.

Kowalski, K. (1985). The impact of chronic grief. *American Journal of Nursing, 85,* 398–399.

Kubler-Ross, E. (1969). *On death and dying.* New York: Macmillan.

Lesher, E. L., & Bergey, K. J. (1988). Bereaved elderly mothers: Changes in health, functional activities, family cohesion, and psychological well-being. *International Journal of Aging and Human Development, 26,* 81–90.

Lincoln, Y. S., & Guba, E. (1985). *Naturalistic inquiry.* Beverly Hills: Sage.

Lindemann, E. (1944). Symptomatology and management of acute grief. *American Journal of Psychiatry, 101,* 141–148.

Martocchio, B. C. (1985). Grief and bereavement. *Nursing Clinics of North America, 20,* 327–341.

Norris, F. H., & Murrell, S. A. (1987). Older adult family stress and adaptation before and after bereavement. *Journal of Gerontology, 42,* 606–612.

Parkes, C. M. (1972). *Bereavement: Studies of grief in adult life.* New York: International Universities.

Parkes, C. M. (1975). Determinants of outcome following bereavement. *Omega, 6,* 303–323.

Parkes, C. M. (1985). Bereavement. *British Journal of Psychiatry, 146,* 11–17.

Paterson, G. W. (1987). Managing grief and bereavement. *Primary Care, 14,* 403–415.

Rodgers, B. L. (1987). *The use and application of concepts in nursing.* Unpublished doctoral dissertation, University of Virginia, Charlottesville.

Rodgers, B. L. (1989a). Concepts, analysis, and the development of nursing knowledge: The evolutionary cycle. *Journal of Advanced Nursing, 14,* 330–335.

Rodgers, B. L. (1989b). Exploring health policy as a concept. *Western Journal of Nursing Research, 11,* 694–702.

Rodgers, B. L., & Cowles, K. V. (1991). The concept of grief: An analysis of classical and contemporary thought. *Death Studies, 15,* 443–458.

Switzer, D. K. (1970). *The dynamics of grief.* New York: Abingdon.

Volkan, V. (1970). Typical findings in pathological grief. *Psychiatric Quarterly, 44,* 231–250.

Worden, J. W. (1985). Bereavement. *Seminars in Oncology, 12,* 472–475.

Zisook, S., & DeVaul, R. (1985). Unresolved grief. *American Journal of Psychoanalysis, 45,* 370–379.

Chapter 8

An Expansion and Elaboration of the Hybrid Model of Concept Development

DONNA SCHWARTZ-BARCOTT AND HESOOK SUZIE KIM

*E*arly in the 1970s, theory development became established as a na-
tional goal in nursing (Meleis, 1985). By 1975, 11 distinct nursing theories
had been published (Walker & Avant, 1988). Simultaneously, nursing educators began experimenting with the incorporation of theories in undergraduate and graduate curricula. The National League for Nursing (1972)
passed a new criterion requiring that curriculum plans be based on conceptual frameworks. The demand for nurses who could teach these theories,
the increasing number of nursing theories, as well as the number of related
nonnursing theories (e.g., stress, communication, coping, systems, and crises
theories) already in the nursing literature made the creation of courses
specific to theory and its application in nursing practice inevitable.

The hybrid model emerged in response to the excitement, exigencies,
and hidden complexities surrounding the development of one such course.
The course that was created at the University of Rhode Island combined a
three-credit theory component with a three-credit practicum. The focus of
the practicum was on selecting, developing, and applying concepts and
theoretical frameworks in specific clinical nursing situations. It quickly became apparent that the excitement over the use of theories in nursing was
not accompanied by an equally developed arsenal of methods for applying
them. There was little, if any, discussion in the nursing literature of how
one was to select from among the various concepts or theories given a
particular clinical problem or situation, or of the possible boundaries or

This chapter is a revised and expanded version of "A hybrid model for concept development." In P. L. Chinn (Ed.), *Nursing research methodology: Issues & implementation* (pp.
91–101), 1986. Reprinted with permission of Aspen Publishers, Inc.

time parameters for applying any one concept or theory. Each theory was seen as appropriate for any nursing care situation or setting. In fact, there seemed to be a rather universal assumption at the time that simply having knowledge of a particular theory was sufficient for its unending application.

An additional difficulty with these early theories was their high degree of abstractness and vagueness. It was not unusual to discover that the central concepts of a theory were lacking adequate definitions or measurements. One manageable way to address these difficulties was to focus attention on the analysis and refinement of individual concepts since they form the basic building blocks of a theory. In so doing, we began looking for an approach that would help ensure that—

1. The concepts selected for analysis would be integral to nursing practice.

2. The literature reviewed would be broad enough to capture the commonalities and extremes in conceptualization and usage of the concept across disciplines.

3. The focus of analysis would be on the essential aspects of definition and measurement.

4. Analysis from the literature review would be tightly integrated with the empirical data being collected in the clinical practicum.

No single approach or literature base addressed all these concerns; thus, an approach (now referred to as the hybrid model of concept development) was created based on knowledge from three bodies of literature, each of which approached concept development in a slightly different manner. These included literature from the philosophy of science (Hempel, 1952; Kaplan, 1964; Nagel, 1961), the sociology of theory construction (Blalock, 1969; Dubin, 1969; Gibbs, 1972; Hage, 1972; Reynolds, 1971) and writings on participant observation—more frequently referred to today as field research (Bogdan & Taylor, 1975; McCall & Simmons, 1969; Pelto, 1970; Schatzman & Strauss, 1973).

The model that was developed interfaces theoretical analysis and empirical observation, with a focus on the essential aspects of definition and measurement. The model involves steps used to identify, analyze, and refine concepts in the initial stage of theory development and is most applicable to applied sciences in general and to nursing specifically. Because the approach draws heavily on insights generated in clinical practice, it is especially useful in studying significant and central phenomena in nursing. Theoretical development based on this model at the initial stage thus can include concepts having both analytical and empirical foundations. The model was first described in Chinn's 1986 edition of *Nursing Research Methodology.* Some of our experience in using the model was presented later in that same year at the Third Annual Nursing Science Colloquium at Boston University (Schwartz-Barcott, 1986). The purpose of this chapter is to integrate these earlier writings with the additions and refinements that have been made to the model over the last five years.

The Hybrid Model

Figure 8–1 presents the major components of the hybrid model. It is composed of three phases: an initial, theoretical phase, a fieldwork phase, and a final, analytical phase. As the label denotes, the initial phase is largely theoretical in nature, although drawing rather heavily on experiences from clinical practice. During this phase, Reynolds's (1971) approach to concept analysis is used to begin the literature search, the analysis of existing definitions, and the selection of a working definition. Reynolds's approach is especially appropriate at this point because of its heavy emphasis on the essential nature of a concept rather than on the defining attributes, properties, antecedents, or consequences of a concept that are of more use after the essential aspect of the concept has been identified. The second phase, which overlaps in time with the first phase, emphasizes the empirical component of the process. In this phase, field research methods are utilized to collect qualitative data for further analysis of the selected concept. The literature review begun in phase one is continued in phase two. Additionally, the literature review serves as an ongoing basis for comparison with data being collected in the field. Schatzman and Strauss's (1973) guide to field research is used directly for the overall structuring and sequencing of steps in this phase. Reynolds's analytical approach helps undergird the collection and analysis of data. Wilson's (1969) analytical approach is brought forth as potentially useful for selecting cases and collecting and analyzing data in

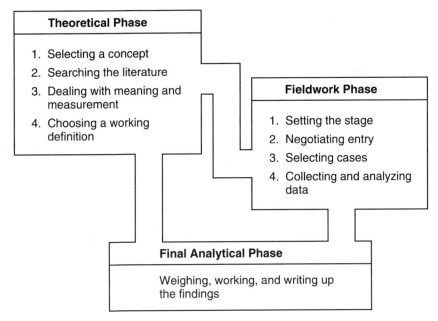

Figure 8–1 A hybrid model of concept development.

the second phase. The third phase includes the final step in interfacing the initial theoretical analysis with insights gained from the empirical obser- vations. Here again Reynolds's and Wilson's analytical approaches help in finalizing the analysis and suggesting possible alterations or refinements of the concept.

The Theoretical Phase

The principal focus in this phase is on developing a foundation for the later phases of in-depth analysis and concept refinement. This includes the se- lection of a concept, initiation of the literature review, a mapping out of essential elements of definition and measurement, and the delineation of a working definition.

SELECTING A CONCEPT

The selection of a concept for study has been approached by nursing schol- ars in various ways. Some authors, such as Brownell (1984), Hogue (1985), Panzarine (1985), and Reed and Leonard (1990), have drawn directly from existing concepts in other disciplines. Others, such as Leininger (1985), Norris (1982), and Rew and Barrow (1987), have drawn on identified but underdeveloped concepts from the nursing literature. Additionally, scholars using grounded theory have generated new concepts directly out of nursing practice or research (Atwood, 1978; Chenitz & Swanson, 1986; Wilson, 1986). Whatever the approach taken, some initial consideration needs to be given to ways of enhancing the probability of selecting a concept relevant to nursing.

The use of an encounter drawn directly from clinical practice can be of great advantage. It can help to guide later theoretical and empirical analyses and, most important, to assure a nursing perspective. Some of the best encounters are those that are unexpected and leave the nurse feeling frus- trated, horrified, angry, embarrassed, or bewildered. For example, a graduate student who was visiting an elderly client in a nursing home for the first time had the following experience:

> *The foyer of the new, modern nursing home was filled with residents. At first glance it seemed to be full of potential hostesses, appropriately attired and positioned to offer a warm welcome to incoming visitors. But, as she entered a step further, moved toward one or two, to nod or smile—expecting in part to be ushered in or at least directed to her client—she discovered distant looks, vacuous smiles and aimless mut- tering.*

The student was surprised to discover that the initial image of social activity and animation among the elderly in the foyer was only a mirage. What was particularly disconcerting and saddening was the lack of human interaction among a group of individuals who appeared to need such interaction.

By filling in details related to the setting, the people involved, and the words exchanged, the investigator can use such an encounter to begin to ferret out a relevant concept. An emphasis on describing the encounter, rather than on trying to explain it, can help avoid premature interpretation. For example, much of the value of the early observations of the elderly group of residents in the foyer of the nursing home would have been lost if the word *"senile"* had been inserted before elderly. *Confusing mutterings* is much more descriptive of the encounter than the single term *confused,* which tends to imply that these individuals were always confused or spent most of their time in a state of confusion. This interpretation would have been erroneous given later observations.

Given a relatively full recording of the encounter, it can be reexamined for possible concepts to be used for labeling, and it can further understanding of the unexpected or problematic aspect of the encounter. The following questions can be used to focus attention on the existing pool of potentially relevant concepts from other disciplines and nursing, thus drawing on two of the approaches mentioned earlier for concept selection. What might be happening here? Is there a single concept, such as withdrawal or noncompliance, that provides a relatively accurate label of the focus of concern? What kind of explanation might a physiologist or psychologist give? How might a sociologist or anthropologist explain this encounter? How might other nurses explain the encounter?

It is not necessary to strike on a single concept immediately. Initially, it is important to consider the wide range of possible scientific concepts or explanations that might help to illuminate this particular encounter. In the encounter with the elderly, one scholar may see indications of disorientation, withdrawal, or some combination of these in the faces and actions of the elderly. Another might see evidence of senility, sensory deprivation, or disengagement. It is not unusual, at this point, to be confronted with a number, even an overabundance, of potential concepts for further examination. In the case just mentioned, five potentially relevant concepts were identified.

There are additional steps that can be taken to focus on a single concept. First, the investigator can begin to delineate concepts that may be more useful as independent variables than as dependent variables. At this point, it is easy to confuse descriptive and explanatory uses of a concept. For example, in the case just mentioned, senility, sensory deprivation, and disengagement were being used primarily as concepts to explain the behavior observed among the elderly in the foyer. Second, the remaining concepts can be arranged by degree of plausibility. The investigator may want to refer back to the initial encounter to review the details in light of the concepts being considered at this point.

In some cases, the investigator still may not be able to draw on any one or two existing concepts directly. Instead, a series of concepts may be identified, none of which seems to capture fully the image of reality that is of interest. In one situation, for example, a nurse was feeling harassed by the picayune, seemingly illogical, and endless demands of a patient who had chronic obstructive lung disease. These demands often were accompanied by abusive language. The patient had a lengthy history of admissions related to his disease and was well known to the staff. No amount of effort on the part of the nursing staff seemed to increase the patient's satisfaction or comfort. As one nurse described it:

> *In cleaning up the bedside table—I moved the Kleenex box—he demanded it be replaced—he wanted it moved another quarter of an inch to the right. The bell would ring once or twice every fifteen minutes. The level of H_2O connected to the O_2 tank was down one-quarter inch, one inch above the level for refill. Mr. J. wanted the water refilled. The function and operation of the water apparatus were explained. Mr. J. nodded in seeming agreement. In five minutes the bell rang again. Mr. J. wanted the H_2O refilled.*

It was not clear whether the nurse was dealing with forgetfulness, autocratism, manipulative behavior, hostility, fear, neurosis, a sense of helplessness, or just open, interpersonal conflict between patient and nurse. All of these concepts seemed to capture an important "reality" in this situation, but at the same time, none seemed to reflect its essence or fullness.

Given this kind of situation, it may be best to go ahead and create a new concept as a basis for tentative exploration in the field setting. Then, later, if an appropriate existing concept emerges, the investigator can simply discard the initial one. It is highly likely that the initial analysis and field data will be useful in examining and refining the existing concept.

SEARCHING THE LITERATURE

A successful review of the literature requires a broad systematic, cross-disciplinary approach. It is important that the investigator begin with a set of questions that will provide an initial direction for the search: What is the essential nature of a concept? How can its essence be defined clearly? How can it be fleshed out so as to enhance its measurability? As these questions suggest, the initial review of the literature needs to be focused on central questions of definition and measurement. The aim is to capture the extremes in conceptualization and usage of the selected concept across disciplines. Later, after the investigator is well into the fieldwork phase, the focus will shift to more subtle elements of definition and measurement. References on integrative research reviews (Cooper, 1984; Ganong, 1987) may be helpful, although their emphasis is often on explanatory relationships derived from empirical research, rather than on definition and measurement of individual concepts across theoretical and empirical literature bases.

DEALING WITH MEANING AND MEASUREMENT

Once a few definitions are in hand, it is helpful to look for major points of contrast and similarity. With a concept such as creativity, the investigator will be confronted with a variety of definitions. For some scholars, creativity is an aspect of cognitive functioning, a way of thinking. For others, it is an intrapersonal and interpersonal process. May (1972) speaks of creativity as an encounter between an intensively conscious human being with his world. But for Rogers (1972), creativity is a "novel relational product growing out of the uniqueness of the individual on the one hand and the materials, events, people or circumstances of his life on the other" (p. 5). Creativity, as a concept, thus is considered as a process of interaction between a person and his or her environment, as a product of interaction, or as an interpersonal process. This type of comparison gives the investigator some idea of the degree of consensus among users of a particular concept and leads to an understanding of what Reynolds (1971) refers to as the degree of inter-subjectivity of meaning.

CHOOSING A WORKING DEFINITION

Once major points of agreement and disagreement have become apparent, a definition is selected or generated for further detailed examination. Selecting a definition that seems congruent with one's initial thoughts will help to maintain a nursing perspective; however, maintaining a tentative posture with respect to a selected definition is necessary if the investigator is to be open-minded in the refinement process.

Fieldwork Phase

The fieldwork phase is aimed at refining a concept by extending and integrating the analysis begun in phase one with ongoing empirical observations initiated in this phase. The approach presented here is a modification of classic participant observation. It includes the basic steps found in any qualitative research that draws heavily on participant observation; setting the stage, negotiating entry, selecting cases, and collecting and analyzing data (Bernard, 1988; Chenitz & Swanson, 1986; Fetterman, 1989; Leininger, 1985; Lofland, 1976; Pelto & Pelto, 1984; Werner & Schoepfle, 1987). The steps in the fieldwork phase, however, differ in scope, focus, and time frame. Classic participant observation studies begin with a broad topical area. Often, the research question itself is not identified until the investigator is well into data collection. The focus generally involves the identification, description, and explanation of several concepts, and the minimum time frame for data collection is usually one year (Bernard, 1988; Keith, 1988; Messerschmidt, 1981; Whyte, 1984). In the hybrid model the focus is on a single concept, identified before the initiation of fieldwork, and on definition and measurement rather than explanation. The minimum time frame for data collection is two and a half to three months.

Schatzman and Strauss (1973) provide an excellent overview of each of the basic steps outlined in Figure 8–1, in *Field Research: Strategies for a Natural Sociology.* The proposed model represents the adaptation of these methods of field research for concept development in nursing. The following discussion highlights techniques that can be used in each step for maintaining the focus on definition and measurement and for incorporating the nursing perspective.

SETTING THE STAGE

The focus in this step is on the selection of a fieldwork site and identification of major questions to guide the fieldwork phase. The selection of a site is somewhat critical to assuring a nursing perspective. By listing the potential range of patient populations or patient care situations in which the concept is expected to be relevant, the investigator can clarify core elements of the concept as well as increase the likely generalizability of the concept within nursing.

For example, in an initial literature review, Testa (1980) found that withdrawal was repeatedly and explicitly linked with elderly people and those who were mentally ill (see Chapter 9). Earlier observations of elderly in nursing homes suggested that withdrawal might occur with considerable frequency in almost any long-term institutionalized patient population. In addition, withdrawal seemed to be more common than indicated in the research on the elderly and the mentally ill populations. At times, it seemed like an almost normal phase—one that most patients pass through in trying to cope with any illness. It appeared, then, that withdrawal may be present with some frequency in a variety of institutional settings, ranging from prisons, mental hospitals, and nursing homes to extended ambulatory care centers and hospices. Withdrawal also may be experienced relatively frequently among the chronically ill and the elderly in noninstitutionalized settings.

Three essential criteria should guide the selection of a population and a setting: (a) the likelihood of frequent observations of the phenomenon under study, (b) the appropriateness of participant observation as a method of gathering empirical data, and (c) the likelihood that the researcher will be able to create and sustain a participant-observation role in the setting. In contrast to earlier and subsequent phases of this model, extensive familiarity with a specific site can act as a strong deterrent in sustaining the participant-observer role. This is depicted well in Benner's (1975) description of her experiences as a nurse-researcher who attempted participant observation in an intensive care unit in which she had previously worked as a staff nurse. She portrayed graphically the difficulties encountered in moving from a participant to an observer role in a setting with which the researcher is very familiar. First, for Benner, her nurse's uniform evoked certain expectations from patients and families but, most importantly, from herself. In one bed, there was a man struggling with a urinal underneath his breakfast tray. Across the hall was an anxious-looking young woman, standing at the foot of the bed of a comatose patient—her eyes searching for help. No other nurses were in sight. Secondly, there were internal pressures she had to accept: the desire to be integrated into the group, the immense discomfort of being treated as an outsider—"the one who does not know the ways of an ICU" (p. 108).

One or two major questions can be used to link the concept with a specific patient population or a setting. For example, the investigator might be interested in the presence of withdrawal among elderly individuals, especially with regard to whether there is a progressive nature to withdrawal. At the same time, it is necessary to deal with the ambiguities inherent in trying to identify any one patient as being *withdrawn.* Questions guiding the fieldwork phase should address (a) the essential defining elements of a concept, (b) the differentiating elements that separate the central concept from similar concepts, and (c) the measurement criteria that may be developed for the concept.

NEGOTIATING ENTRY

It is easy to disregard the subtleties of gaining access and legitimation to the selected population or setting demands until it is too late. In *Field Research,* Schatzman and Strauss (1973) cover the intricacy and complexity of this type of negotiation in much detail—especially as it applies to formal and highly complex organizations, such as a hospital. Many additional discussions of entry-level issues and techniques can be found in the large volume of writings that are currently available on the relational and personal processes of fieldwork (see for example, Agar, 1980; Ellen, 1984; Emerson, 1983; Wax, 1986; Whyte, 1984; and Zola, 1983 in the sociological and anthropological literature and Davis, 1986; Evaneshko, 1985; Field, 1989; and Wilson, 1982 in the nursing literature).

SELECTING CASES

Decisions regarding with whom the investigator should speak and how to focus observations in the field depend on the unit of analysis under study and the degree of clarity and intersubjectivity found in the initial review of literature. The unit of analysis depends on the concept. It most likely would be at the individual level for a study of withdrawal among the elderly or at the dyad level for a study of the use of touch among couples attending Lamaze classes. Other concepts that may be studied at the dyad level include empathy, attraction, and anger. Empathy and anger are also illustrative of concepts that may be studied at multiple levels. A small group could be a unit of analysis, if the investigator focused on empathetic interaction among group members. An entire unit, such as a floor in a nursing home, might be the unit of analysis if the presence of multiple patient roles and their patterns of interaction were of interest. As the investigator moves from a small group to a larger unit of analysis, however, more time is needed in order to gain adequate baseline knowledge of and familiarity with the group or unit under study.

A large number of cases is unnecessary and undesirable with this model of concept development. Three to six individuals, three or four dyads, one or two groups, and one floor or ward are more appropriate, since this enhances the possibility of frequent, repeated contact. Single encounters do not allow sufficient time for reflecting and probing. The selection of any one individual, couple, group, or floor will depend on the degree of definitional clarity gained in the theoretical phase. If the essential features of the concept are relatively clear, one or two indicators can serve as a basis for selection.

If the essential features of the concept are not clear and no indicators are apparent, Wilson's (1969) typology for concept analysis can be used as a basis for selection. This typology begins with the *model* case—one that absolutely reflects an instance of the concept. As Wilson notes, this is an instance in which we hear ourselves saying, "Well, if that isn't an example of so-and-so, then nothing is" (p. 28). Second is the *contrary* case, which according to Wilson represents a case that is absolutely not an instance of the concept: "Well, whatever so-and-so is, that certainly isn't an instance of it" (p. 29). Third is the *borderline* case. It appears as the "odd or queer" case (p. 31) and it helps highlight elements that make for a "true" case. The typology ends with the *related* case, which helps to clarify the central concept by identifying the criteria for a related concept.

The following excerpt from St. Angelo's (1983) observations of patient-nurse interactions in an emergency room provides an example of a model case of bonding. St. Angelo wondered if the concept of bonding (taken from the infant-mother bonding literature) might also be relevant to certain, rather "special" adult-nurse encounters that sometimes occur in the emergency room (ER).

The Model Case. *The emergency room doors opened. The rescue workers brought in a 55-year-old man with gasoline burns on his face, neck and chest. His lawnmower had exploded. He was conscious and had a saline-soaked drape on his face to cool the burns. Sue, the nurse, immediately took Mr. G.'s hand and told him her name and that she would be taking care of him. "I'm going to leave the drape on your face to cool the burns. Your chest is burned and I need to get these clothes off of you. Do you mind if I cut them?" Mr. G. replied, "Honey, you do anything you have to." Sue went on to tell Mr. G. that she was also going to have to draw some blood, start an intravenous, and that the doctor would be putting a Foley catheter into his bladder because of the need to monitor all the fluids going in and out of his body. Mr. G. jokingly said to Sue: "OK, but tell the doctor to cover me up—I'm shy." Sue told Bob not to worry as she drew the curtains around him and "whenever we aren't working on you we'll keep you covered. There's only me, another nurse and the doctor here."*

Sue began to do the procedures necessary, explaining everything to Mr. G. as she went along. He asked her questions about the extent of his burns and about the other people at the scene. She answered as she worked. At one point Mr. G. jokingly said: "Hey Sue, what does my face look like? I hope I'm not going to be an ugly duckling." Sue came to the bedside, took his hand and spoke quietly at Mr. G.'s ear level: "Bob, you have some blisters on your face and I'm leaving the wet drape on so it will cool the area. Your eyelids might swell a little but it will go down in a couple of days. We have an excellent plastic surgeon coming in and he will debride the burns and start cleaning them with a special cream. You should have minimal to no scarring." In a more serious tone Mr. G. responded: "Well, I was just wondering . . . I have a heavy date with my wife for New Year's Eve."

The plastic surgeon was delayed in getting to the ER so there was a long waiting period. Sue stayed with Mr. G. during this time doing paper work at his bedside. She contacted family, offered pain medication prn and fed Mr. G. ice chips. The drape remained on Mr. G.'s face the entire time. When Sue transferred Mr. G. to a room on the surgical unit, Sue placed her hand on Mr. G.'s forehead and jokingly said: "Well, you took so much of my time today, Bob, that it's almost time for me to go home." Mr. G. responded: "Well, you turned out to be a swell date, Sue. We'll have to do this again sometime. Maybe next time I'll at least be able to see your face."

Next Saturday morning Sue went up on the floor to visit Mr. G. He was sitting up eating breakfast. His face had silvadene cream on it but his eyes were exposed. His lids were slightly swollen but they were open. Sue went into the room, smiled and said hello to Bob. He said hello but appeared hesitant as if he didn't know her. Sue went to the bedside and said: "Bob, my name is Sue. I took care of you in the emergency department on Thursday." Bob took Sue's hand and smiled: "Honey, I don't recognize you but I'd know that voice anywhere." (pp. 10–11)

Later, another excerpt from St. Angelo's observation (1983), was selected as a contrary case. Whatever was going on between this nurse and patient, it clearly was not an instance of bonding.

The Contrary Case. *An 87-year-old man was wheeled into the ER. He had come from a local nursing home. On his right shoulder and scapular area was a large abscess. He was to meet his private physician for an incision and drainage of the abscess. The nurse, Peter, introduced himself to Mr. E., who was hard of hearing. Mr. E. was oriented to person and place but displayed some confusion as to time. Peter took Mr. E.'s vital signs and tried to obtain a patient history but Mr. E. was a poor historian. Peter sat at the desk and obtained the needed information from the transfer record. He returned to Mr. E. to make sure he was warm and safe. Peter then went about his other duties while waiting for the private physician to arrive. He periodically checked back with Mr. E. to see if there was anything he needed and to reassure him that the doctor would be coming. Mr. E. never asked for anything but always acknowledged Peter's orientation as to why he was waiting. The doctor arrived one hour later without apology. Peter immediately began to set up the anticipated equipment. He helped Mr. E. turn on his side. Peter then bent over, looked Mr. E. in the eyes and explained what would happen. "The doctor is going to wash your back with medicine and then he's going to put some medicine in your upper back to make it numb. You have to hold still." Mr. E. acknowledged Peter's comments with an "OK." The doctor proceeded with the procedure while Peter assisted. When the incision was made, a large amount of foul smelling drainage escaped. Everyone in the immediate area made facial expressions which indicated their awareness of the offensive odor. Mr. E. never said a word. Peter occasionally bent over to look at Mr. E. to ask how he was doing. Mr. E. would always respond, "OK." The incision was packed by the doctor and Peter applied a bulky dressing. Peter asked Mr. E. if he had any pain. Mr. E. did not comment. Peter asked again but a little louder. This time Mr. E. said "a little." Peter said he would get him some pain medication.*

Later, Peter returned with the medication. He told Mr. E. that he would call the ambulance to take Mr. E. back to the nursing home. Peter called the home to review all the doctor's orders with the nurse who would be caring for Mr. E. He later found out that the ambulance would be delayed. He called the kitchen and ordered a lunch tray for Mr. E. Peter explained the situation to Mr. E. and assisted him with the lunch tray. (pp. 1914–1915)

Both of these encounters were selected for more intensive case work. Later, during the analysis phase, the cases were used to help identify essential aspects of bonding by eliminating the unessential features.

COLLECTING AND ANALYZING THE DATA

Schatzman and Strauss's (1973) notation system for collecting, recording, and analyzing fieldwork data is particularly well suited for concept analysis and refinement. This system utilizes a combination of participant observation augmented with periodic in-depth interviews. It facilitates multiple observations and in-depth reflection as well as probing dialogue with participants over time. Although there are several more recent publications on analyzing qualitative data (Bernard, 1988; Miles & Huberman, 1984; Strauss, 1987), this system is especially helpful in defining and measuring single concepts. More recent techniques tend to focus on the development of theoretical hypotheses or propositions, which often shifts the focus from definition and measurement to explanation.

The notation system includes observational notes (ON), theoretical notes (TN), and methodological notes (MN) that guide the researcher into possible analytic distinctions at the point of recording. The ON "are statements bearing upon events experienced principally through watching and listening. They contain as little interpretation as possible, and are as reliable as the observer can construct them" (Schatzman & Strauss, 1973, pp. 94–108). This is the who, what, when, where, and how of the phenomenon and identifies who said or did what under what circumstances. Quotation marks can be used to identify the exact words, phrases, or sentences that occurred in any one conversation. Otherwise, an apostrophe can be used for less accurate quoting or for simply paraphrasing. The TN is used to go beyond the "facts." The investigator can consciously interpret, infer, or speculate about the possible meaning of the observations. In the hybrid model, one can use the TN for bringing in definitions and measurements from the literature for comparing and contrasting with the data just described in the ON. The investigator's instructions to himself or herself are included under MN. This notation system encourages free-flowing yet systematic recording and organizing of the data. It makes for easy retrieval of key observations and is conducive to continual analysis and reflection.

Analyzing the Data. As is apparent from the notation system, data collection plunges the investigator into the analysis phase. Collection and analysis of data go on concurrently with every other step under the rubric of the TN. Nevertheless, about one half to three fourths of the way through the fieldwork phase, the investigator needs to begin to pull out and organize the data that are most relevant to the concept. Wilson's (1969) typology of cases can be helpful here. This can then serve as a basis for refocusing ongoing field observations and for more focused, in-depth probing as one moves through the latter half of this phase.

Mr. G. was the *model* case described earlier. He came into the ER with face, neck, and chest burns from a lawnmower accident. St. Angelo (1983) first compared the behavioral indicators of bonding (for example, nonprocedural touch; frequent, sustained eye contact; a "caring" tone of voice) that had emerged in the literature review of mother-infant bonding, with her own field observations:

> *In this case, I saw indicators of touch. Hand-holding and gentle touch during the procedure were common. Also, when we brought Bob to his room, Sue put her hand on Bob's forehead as if to soothe him. There was absolutely no eye contact during this encounter which took about 5½ hours. Sue's tone of voice was very different from what I would have anticipated. Yet, it seemed to be very effective. She used a calm, confident tone of voice mixed with a joking attitude. There was indirect acknowledgement of but almost no direct reflection of Sue's or the patient's feelings. The patient's voice was initially shaky, then mixed with a joking attitude. (p. 14)*

Touch, either procedural or nonprocedural, may reflect an essential element in patient-nurse bonding just as it does in mother-infant bonding. Sustained eye contact was not possible in this case because of the nature of the patient's injury. However, contrary to the literature, the lack of eye contact suggested that bonding can take place in the absence of such contact. Additionally, measurement problems became abundantly clear. St. Angelo struggled to judge whether a nurse's tone of voice demonstrated a *caring* quality.

Next, the data are reexamined to see if there are any *contrary* cases. These can be compared with model cases to highlight that which is distinctive to the latter. The following is an excerpt from St. Angelo's analysis of the contrary case presented earlier between the ER nurse, Peter, and Mr. E., an 87-year-old resident of a local nursing home who had come to the ER with a large abscess on his shoulder.

> *I noticed that Peter did not use touch at any time other than to carry out a procedure. Yet, his touch was gentle, purposeful and appeared therapeutic. At first I interpreted this negatively but further searching of the literature suggested another possible view. I was interpreting touch (significant touch) to be anything other than procedural touch, but is that true? Peter's touch during procedures was always gentle. I began to equate this with the mother-infant literature and my own life experiences. After all, a mother's touch during diaper change is considered to be loving and caring. Sundeen, Stuart, Rankin, and Cohen (1976) state that the "use of touch in nursing goes beyond that which is necessary to attend to the client's personal physical needs. The manner in which the person is touched and the attitude of the nurse who is touching can convey a message of caring while physical needs are met" (p. 103). This literature changed my entire focus on Peter's care. Still I did not feel that this reflected "bonding." Instead, I would call it "caring." (pp 23–24)*

Earlier the term *bonding* was used to describe the special binding relationship that emerged between Sue and Bob. It seems completely missing in the encounter between Peter and Mr. E., even though Peter's touch denotes an element of caring. Thus, it may be that caring can occur without bonding taking place. In fact, there may be two separate or intertwining concepts in these situations: caring and bonding. Caring may be a necessary but not a sufficient component of bonding. Or, caring may be a separate but closely related concept. At the same time, this stage of analysis suggested the need to refocus attention on what is it that seems so unique to adult bonding. How can this kind of special interpersonal exchange in which each individual somehow becomes wedded to the other be "put into words?"

In the *borderline case,* it is not clear whether the concept applies. As Wilson (1969) notes, "by seeing what makes these cases 'odd or queer,' we come to see why the 'true' cases are not odd or queer" (p. 31) or, in other words, what makes them true cases. An example of a borderline case was not encountered in St. Angelo's field observations of bonding. A borderline case was present, however, in Robert's (1982) field study of empathy among members in a sharing and caring group, namely, the Compassionate Friends, a group composed mainly of bereaved parents.

At the December meeting, the group discussion centered around the upcoming holidays. A discussion about holiday tradition revealed a similarity between Pat and Betty; following that a significant interchange between these two women occurred. Pat was discussing her feelings regarding Christmas without her son. Betty, who appeared to have been listening intently, responded by talking about her own emotional experiences and feelings regarding the holiday. As Betty spoke, Pat remained seated on the edge of her chair, leaning towards Betty and maintaining eye contact. When Betty paused, Pat proceeded to finish the story she had previously started, her voice revealing the intensity of her feelings. This "conversation" continued as both women verbally expressed their feelings. Neither one of them responded to the feelings expressed by the other, but instead focused on their own emotional experience which seemed similar. The rest of the group remained attentive and seemingly involved with the dialogue. I sensed a feeling of closeness between Pat and Betty following this interaction (pp. 13–14).

Pat and Betty were intensely engaged in conversation in this example. Yet, neither one acknowledged or responded directly to the specifics of what the other said. At the same time, however, both women seemed to experience the interaction as positive and helpful. What made this case "odd or queer," in terms of empathy, was the failure of either party to react to the specific feelings being expressed by the other, although each responded to the other by sharing a similar experience or feeling. This analysis later led Roberts (1982) to propose three different degrees or levels of empathy:

Level one: *Individuals respond to each other by sharing a similar experience or emotion, but do not react to the specific feelings being expressed by the other.*

Level two: *One individual (the empathizer) recognizes that the feelings being expressed belong to the other. The empathizer may begin to respond to the feelings being expressed by the other.*

Level three: *The empathizer begins to feel, think, and act like the other, mirroring his or her emotion. At the same time, however, he or she maintains a clear sense of self and personal identity (pp. 15–16).*

Here, the odd case actually became incorporated within the concept as a minimal level indicator of empathy. Secondly, in constructing these levels, Roberts was able to move the measurement of empathy from a nominal to an ordinal level.

Another way of analyzing the data is to look for what Wilson (1969) called the *related* case: one which reflects a concept similar to the one under study. Often, this kind of case appears serendipitously. Sometimes, the investigator can be looking at a focal concept and discover another concept. Wilson suggests that the investigator can clarify the criteria for applying the related concept and may, in turn, be able to "get clear" more easily about the original concept. Here is an example from St. Angelo's (1983) study on patient-nurse bonding in an emergency room setting.

A 36-year-old female was wheeled into the ER by the triage nurse. She was obese and stated that she had MS (multiple sclerosis). She was presently having urological problems for which the physician inserted a Foley catheter until further testing and possible surgery could be done. The Foley catheter had fallen out and the client wanted the catheter replaced. The nurse helped undress the client and inserted the catheter. During this time, the client shared that she had once weighed about 500 lbs and now weighed 350 lbs. She attributed the excessive weight gain to prednisone which she took for the MS. The client had poor personal hygiene and the body odor was difficult to deal with in such close quarters. Her perineal area was also in need of good hygiene. During the actual insertion of the catheter, the nurse never looked at the client; however, she maintained the conversation throughout the procedure. The nurse spoke with inflections and a tone of voice which demonstrated a warmth and caring. She utilized therapeutic reflective communication techniques and seemed to have a good understanding of the client's situation and feelings. At one point the client commented that she really hoped the catheter would be taken out soon and that the doctor would take care of this problem. The nurse responded: "You

*really feel gypped, don't you?" To this, the client paused and then said:
"Yeah—I'm supposed to be getting married soon and this is making
things hard on me—pause—I don't want to be left out." The nurse
commented: "And I suppose your doctor really doesn't understand that."
The client ended this exchange with, "Well, I guess not"—pause—"the
tests will be done soon to see if I have a blockage . . ."*

*In this example, there was no eye contact, no touching other than
procedural or purposeful, but the tone of voice was unique. The nurse
used a concerned tone of voice with a lot of inflections and excellent
reflective techniques. St. Angelo interpreted the nurse's communications
as a taking in, digesting and giving back of an understanding of the
client, which the client validated in her responses. The nurse was attempting to communicate to the client that her ideas, feelings, and so
on, were the ones that are important, not those of the nurses or others.*

*As the nurse mentioned in the staff conference, she had some diffi-
culty maintaining her professionalism because of the body odor. St.
Angelo saw a lot of energy being used in this case. It took energy to
maintain professionalism in a difficult situation. It took energy to care
for someone the nurse found to be offensive and still utilize a therapeutic communication. Also, it is not clear why the nurse did not look
at the client during her care. Were there some personal feelings related
to the client's age (close to the nurse's) and her pending marriage in
spite of her obesity and her disease, that were affecting the nurse? Obese
women with crippling disease and urinary tract problems in our society
are not usually portrayed as sexual beings. Yet, the nurse was able to
overcome most of these aspects to the best of her ability by providing
the client with what might most accurately be called empathy. (pp.
16–17)*

Thus, in looking for evidence of bonding, St. Angelo uncovered empathy.
The bonding indicator of touch was not present, although the student saw
a "caring" quality in the tone of voice. But, more important in this analysis
was the description of the nurse's inherent dislike of the patient. It took a
lot of energy and concentration for the nurse to keep this element from
interfering with the care she felt the patient needed. It would seem, then,
that a mutual liking and attraction needs to emerge between the patient
and the nurse, in the context of the nurse's touch and caring, in order for
bonding to take place. And, it is perhaps this special mutual attraction that
best characterizes the unique aspect of a bonding relationship.

Final Analytical Phase

During the analytical phase, the investigator steps back from the intensity
and details of the fieldwork and reexamines the findings in light of the initial
focus of interest. The following questions may be asked in this phase:

- How much is the concept applicable and important to nursing?
- Does the initial selection of the concept seem justified?
- To what extent do the review of literature, theoretical analysis, and empirical findings support the presence and frequency of this concept within the population selected for empirical study?

For example, Testa's (1980) fieldwork with withdrawal tended to support the presence and importance of psychosocial withdrawal among residents in a nursing home setting. At the same time, the fieldwork suggested that, although the phenomenon existed frequently, withdrawal was not necessarily inherent in the adjustment process. In addition, the review of the literature and empirical findings altered an earlier perception of withdrawal as a predominantly negative process. It became apparent that withdrawal can be a positive factor by providing a "time-out" period for energy renewal and in maintaining one's self-dignity as well as gaining some control over the immediate environment, even when that environment reflects the dictates of a total institution.

At other times, the investigator may be less convinced of the relevance of a concept after fieldwork than he or she was before. Sometimes it is not so much that the findings do not support the existence of a particular concept as it is that a new concept or reformulation of the initial idea emerges out of the empirical observations and analysis. For example, Hassma (1979) was surprised to find little empirical support for the presence and importance of denial among repeat heart attack victims. She had expected to encounter a high level of denial among patients who showed a substantial lag period between the appearance of symptoms and hospitalization. Instead, Hassma found that difficulties in the process of "differential diagnosis," by patients, families, and in some cases physicians, was more a factor in producing a significant lag period than was the denial of symptoms.

Sometimes, it is not so much that the findings do not support the existence of a particular concept as it is that a new concept or reformulation of the initial idea emerges out of the empirical observations and analysis. For example, Janicki (1981) began fieldwork with a focus on the "mental suffering" of patients in the terminal phase of an illness, usually cancer. As she became more and more precise in the description of these patients' sufferings, the term *anguish* began to emerge as a more accurate label of the phenomenon she was observing.

If the importance of the initial concept was supported, then the next step is to reconsider the findings in light of the concept's definition and measurability. The investigator may want to begin by going back to the initial, tentative definitions and the listing of key elements in, and the analysis of, these definitions. At this stage, the investigator is asking, How do the definitions compare and contrast with the empirical findings? It may be that, at this point, one definition stands out as more useful than another. For example, Reilly (1982) found that creativity, in the context of nursing home residents, was far more an "active life process," involving one's entire being, than it was predominantly an activity of the mind. She also began to see an association between an individual's level of adjustment and the person's level of creativity. Those who adjusted exceedingly well seemed to actively remold the nursing home. Sometimes this remolding included the rearrangement of furniture in their rooms. Other times it occurred on a larger scale, such as the negotiation of a new role—that is, mailman or gardener—within the institutional setting. Whichever the case, for those who did very well, the adjustment was not simply passive acceptance of a given environment but a seeking out and revamping of that environment.

In another case, the empirical findings may lead to a redefinition of a concept or refinements in an existing definition. Testa (1980) concluded that psychosocial withdrawal needed to be separated explicitly from physical withdrawal. Also, the former concept needed to be redefined in terms of a process rather than as simply a symptom of something else or as a solitary state. Additionally, withdrawal needed to be reconceived as a social-psychological process that could range along a continuum of normality and not be limited to an abnormal, purely intrapsychic experience.

Yet, in other cases, it may be a matter of making explicit what has been implicit in the literature. Roberts (1982) defined *empathy* as an active process in which an individual senses another's emotional state, identifies with this state unconsciously or consciously, and reacts to the state, which results in a sharing of feelings. The importance of this definition was in making the implicit explicit. Additionally, in defining empathy in this way, it became possible to differentiate empathy from imitative behavior—an important distinction not included in earlier definitions.

Empirical findings also may lead to the recommendation of a new way of measuring a concept or to suggestions for refinements in existing measures. For example, Testa (1980) was able to begin operationalizing *withdrawal* by identifying a complex of physical, social, and emotional indicators. And, differing levels of severity were identified, which allowed for measurement at the categorical level. Her empirical findings lend support to these beginning efforts at measuring withdrawal.

Sometimes, the empirical findings may simply raise the need for different indicators, given the lack of support for existing ones. To some extent, this was one of the results of St. Angelo's work on adult bonding. The indicators from the mother-infant bonding literature (continuous eye contact, non-procedural touch, and tone of voice) were just not comprehensive or germane enough to adult-adult relationships of this nature. Instead, it seemed that the investigator needed to look more closely at some form of subjective indicator, or a mixture of these more objective ones, with one or two more subjective indicators.

WRITING UP THE FINDINGS

Reporting the results of a hybrid model analysis requires the integration of two separate writing traditions, concept analysis and fieldwork. The best single approach to integrating these traditions, to date, has been to frame the introduction and initial review of the literature in accord with the classic format of concept analysis and then draw on writing styles used in fieldwork to present and integrate the empirical observations with the literature review.

Textbooks and writings on concept development in the social sciences and in nursing seldom address the various techniques and formats used to write up a concept analysis (Bulmer, 1984; Chinn & Jacobs, 1983; Norris, 1982; Sartori, 1984; Walker & Avant, 1988; Wilson, 1969). In general, the author must use examples, such as those provided by Norris (1982), Kim (1983), Bertman and Krant (1977) and Gardner (1979). Kim (1983) presented two examples of mini-analyses of the concepts of restlessness and compliance that aligned well with the emphasis on definition and measurement found in the hybrid model. In each analysis, Kim moved from a discussion of definitions across diverse bodies of literature to differentiation of the concept from other similar concepts (like Wilson's borderline or related concepts), to operationalization, and lastly to possible relationships with other concepts. In addition there is a need to begin with a discussion of the importance and relevance of the concept in nursing.

In writing up the empirical findings, the investigator has to consider the same questions facing any researcher in reporting a study involving field-work data: Who will the audience, or reader, be? What should the timing and pacing of the writing process be? How long should the manuscript be? Which details of methodology should be included? How should credibility be established? What facts or interpretations can ethically be made public? Early textbooks on participant observation addressed these issues in detail (see, for example, Bogdan & Taylor, 1975; Lofland & Lofland, 1984; McCall & Simmons, 1969; Schatzman & Strauss, 1973). In addition, Taylor and Bogdan (1984) identified seven basic points of methodology (for example, time and length of study and researcher's frame of mind) that serve as a useful checklist of content not to be forgotten. Lofland and Lofland's (1984) depiction of the necessary stages involved in writing a fieldwork report (from withdrawal and contemplation to the agony of omitting material and the creating of a serious outline) help the author anticipate the time and skills necessary for this type of writing.

More recent writings on participant observation have suggested that the presentation also needs to reflect the underlying purpose and the particular fieldwork approach taken in the study, for example, Lofland's (1976) strategic interaction orientation, Spradley's (1980) ethnographic approach, and Glaser's (1978) and Strauss's (1987) grounded theory methodology. Perhaps the model most closely approximating the kind of participant observation used in the hybrid model is grounded theory. The investigator, however, must keep in mind that the focus in grounded theory is on categorizing key concepts and explicating theoretical relationships, rather than on defining and measuring these concepts. On the horizon, investigators can expect to find an even wider range of considerations and styles for writing up fieldwork, as the recent debates and efforts of anthropologists to incorporate more humanistic and reflexive aspects of fieldwork into the reports themselves become known (for example, see Danforth, 1989; Denzin, 1989; Geertz, 1988; and Van Maanen, 1988).

Uses of the Hybrid Model to Date

Over the last 13 years, the hybrid model has been applied in a relatively wide variety of nursing care settings. Over 70 concepts have been examined. The concepts we have examined to date are shown in Tables 8–1 and 8–2, in order to give an idea of the range and nature of these concepts. Concepts that relate to the client-nurse domain are shown in Table 8–1. These are concepts that characterize in some way the nature of client-nurse interactions.

The concepts seemed to form into certain clusters. For example, some, such as caring, mutuality, bonding, and friendship, tend to reflect more the quality of an interaction than the fundamental process or the central focus of an interaction. In contrast, concepts of power and exchange relate to central processes of the interaction itself. And concepts such as presence, touch, empathy and advocacy are more narrowly focused on the quality of the nurse's action. Examples of concepts that relate more exclusively to the client domain are given in Table 8–2. Here, there is less of an apparent clustering among concepts. Kim's (1983) scheme for categorizing phenomena in the client domain provides a beginning basis for clustering the concepts examined to date. The three relevant categories in this scheme include (a) essentialist concepts that refer to "phenomena present in the client as essential characteristics and processes of human nature," (b) problematic concepts that refer to "phenomena present in human beings as pathological or abnormal deviations from normal patternings" and (c) health care experiential concepts that refer to "phenomena that arise from people's experiences in the health care system" (p. 43).

To date, the model has been useful in at least four ways. First, it has been helpful in giving some initial idea about the existence, frequency, and potential importance of any one concept in a given patient care setting. Each time we have used the model we have come away with a rather solid notion of the adequacy or inadequacy of existing definitions and possible approaches to measurability. For example, the results of one study suggested that the concept of independence may be unduly limited to an individual's physical ability to carry out a manual task. For example, given current

Table 8–1	*Client-Nurse Domain*

Concepts Reflecting the Character of an Interaction
Caring

Mutuality

Bonding

Therapeutic alliance

Attachment

Friendship

Concepts Characterizing Subprocesses Underlying or Forming the Focus of an Interaction
Central Process
Power

Exchange

Subprocesses
Independence/dependence/interdependence

Information seeking

Decision making

Self-disclosure

Trust

Concepts Reflecting Some Aspect of Actions of Nurse
Presence

Touch

Affective sensitivity

Empathy

Advocacy

Validation

---

definitions, the following two individuals would be considered extremely dependent—a notion we found difficult to comprehend: (1) a paralyzed elderly client capable of orchestrating an array of personal services to maintain her living quarters in a private apartment complex and (2) a kidney dialysis patient able to supervise, instruct, and support his wife's performance of the daily dialysis routines.

Secondly, the shortened time frame of the hybrid model has facilitated multiple analyses of single concepts. These additional analyses have been especially helpful in (1) examining a concept's relevancy and centrality across nursing settings and (b) separating the essential aspects of a concept

Table 8–2	*Client Domain*

Essentialist Concepts

Relaxation	Fatalism
Dying	Control
Creativity	Adaptation
Independence	Self-care
Coping	Territoriality
Problem solving	Personal space
Information seeking	Self-esteem
Decision making	Body image
Definition of the situation	Connectedness
Temperament	Autonomy
Hope	Parenting
Faith	Support

Problematic Concepts

Pain	Chronic sorrow
Fatigue	Helplessness
Restlessness	Panic
Suffering	Boredom
Memory loss	Loneliness
Obesity	Submission
Delayed recovery	Withdrawal
Homelessness	Isolation
Masking behavior	Anomie
Denial	Alienation
Fear	Negligence
Anguish	Stigmatization

Health Care Experiential Concepts

Noncompliance

Stigma

Separation anxiety

from those that systematically vary across clinical settings and specialty areas. For example, in the fieldwork phases of three analyses, we found fear to be a consistently important and frequent phenomenon. This is in marked contrast to the heavy emphasis placed on anxiety in the nursing literature.

The fieldwork phases of these analyses dealt with the fear experienced by women in anticipation of labor and delivery (Hightower, 1979), patients waiting for hospitalization for cardiac surgery (Seidler, 1981), and by myocardial infarction patients during hospital and posthospital phases of recovery (Amato-Vealey, 1987). In each setting, the essential quality of fear as an emotional response to a consciously recognized and external threat of danger and its distinctiveness from anxiety was confirmed. At the same time, the specific content, timing, and duration of the fear varied according to the event around which the fear centered.

Additionally, multiple analyses have helped to identify situations where nurses may mistakenly be using a single concept (for example, withdrawal) to label what are actually two distinct phenomena, such as psychosocial withdrawal as opposed to physical, or substance, withdrawal. A similar situation seems to be occurring with the concept of empathy. Nurses may need to consider separating clinical empathy, as a conscious and cognitive-based nursing intervention, from the more spontaneous and experientially based empathy seen among patients, such as that described earlier in Roberts's (1982) work with two self-help groups (Dalton, 1989).

A third and unintentional outcome of the fieldwork phase of the model has been the illumination of both problematic and nonproblematic consequences of a given phenomenon. A good example of this is seen in Verhulst's work on withdrawal, which is presented in the next chapter. Studies such as this provide important baseline information for developing nursing diagnoses.

A fourth unexpected result of many of the concept analyses completed to date has been the identification of clusters of concepts that appear to be interrelated (for example, problem solving, decision making and compliance, or isolation, loneliness, and social support). This has prompted work on a second model (The Cluster Differentiation Model), which is currently being developed by the authors. It is aimed at identifying the relationships among a small cluster of concepts as a step toward explanation and the identification of relational statements. There appears to be a need for a sequence of steps (or models) that incorporate traditional techniques of theory development with modified and highly focused fieldwork methods aimed at enhancing inductive theory development in nursing.

REFERENCES

Agar, M. (1980). *The professional stranger: An informal introduction to ethnography.* New York: Academic.

Amato-Vealey, E. (1987). A concept analysis of fear as experienced by myocardial infarct patients. Unpublished manuscript. University of Rhode Island, Kingston, RI.

Atwood, J. R. (1978). The phenomenon of selective neglect. In E. Bauwens (Ed.), *The anthropology of health* (pp. 192–200). St. Louis: Mosby.

Benner, P. (1975). Nurses in the intensive care unit. In M. Z. Davis, M. Kramer, & A. L. Strauss (Eds.), *Nurses in practice: A perspective on work environments* (pp. 106-128). St. Louis: Mosby.

Bernard, R. H. (1988). *Research methods in cultural anthropology.* Newbury Park, Calif: Sage.

Bertman, S., & Krant, M. J. (1977). To know of suffering and the teaching of empathy. *Social Science and Medicine, 1,* 53–61.

Blalock, H. M. (1969). *Theory construction: From verbal to mathematical formulations.* Englewood Cliffs, NJ: Prentice-Hall.

Bogdan, R., & Taylor, S. J. (1975). *Introduction to qualitative research methods.* New York: John Wiley & Sons.

Brownell, M. J. (1984). The concept of crisis: Its utility for nursing. *Advances in Nursing Science, 6*(4), 10–21.

Bulmer, M. (1984). Concepts in the analysis of qualitative data. In M. Bulmer (Ed.), *Sociological research methods* (pp. 241–262). New Brunswick, NJ: Transaction Books.

Chenitz, W. C., & Swanson, J. M. (1986). *From practice to grounded theory: Qualitative research in nursing.* Reading, Mass: Addison-Wesley.

Chinn, P. L., & Jacobs, M. K. (1983). *Theory and nursing: A systematic approach.* St. Louis: Mosby.

Chinn, P. L. (1986). *Nursing research methodology: Issues and implementations.* Rockville, Md: Aspen.

Cooper, H. M. (1984). *The integrative research review: A systematic approach.* Beverly Hills: Sage.

Dalton, J. (1989). Empathy, social support and caring: A cluster analysis. Unpublished manuscript. University of Rhode Island, Kingston, RI.

Danforth, L. M. (1989). *Firewalking and religious healing.* Princeton, NJ: Princeton University Press.

Davis, M. Z. (1986). Observation in natural settings. In W. C. Chenitz & J. M. Swanson (Eds.), *From practice to grounded theory: Qualitative research in nursing* (pp 48–65). Reading, Mass: Addison-Wesley.

Denzin, N. (1989). Review symposium on field methods. *Journal of Contemporary Ethnography, 18*(1), 89–109.

Dubin, R. (1969). *Theory building: A practical guide to the construction and testing of theoretical models.* New York: Free Press.

Ellen, R. F. (1984). *Ethnographic research: A guide to general conduct.* New York: Academic Press.

Emerson, R. M. (1983). *Contemporary field research: A collection of readings.* Boston: Little, Brown.

Evaneshko, V. (1985). Entrée strategies for nursing field research studies. In M. M. Leininger (Ed.), *Qualitative research methods in nursing* (pp. 133–148). New York: Grune & Stratton.

Fetterman, D. M. (1989). *Ethnography: Step by step.* Newbury Park, Calif: Sage.

Field, P. A. (1989). Doing fieldwork in your own culture. In J. M. Morse (Ed.), *Qualitative nursing research: A contemporary dialogue* (pp. 79–91). Rockville, Md: Aspen.

Ganong, L. H. (1987). Integrative reviews of nursing research. *Research in Nursing and Health, 10,* 1–11.

Gardner, K. (1979). Supportive nursing: A critical review of the literature. *Journal of Psychiatric Nursing and Mental Health Services, 17*(10), 10–16.

Geertz, C. (1988). *Works and lives: The anthropologist as author.* Palo Alto, Calif: Stanford University Press.

Gibbs, J. (1972). *Sociological theory construction.* Hinsdale, Ill: Dryden Press.

Glaser, B. G. (1978). *Theoretical sensitivity: Advances in the methodology of grounded theory.* Mill Valley, Calif: The Sociology Press.

Hage, J. (1972). *Techniques and problems of theory construction in sociology.* New York: John Wiley & Sons.

Hassma, J. (1979). A concept analysis of denial. Unpublished manuscript. University of Rhode Island, Kingston, RI.

Hempel, C. G. (1952). *Fundamentals of concept formation in empirical science.* Chicago: University of Chicago Press.

Hightower, A. (1979). A concept analysis of fear in the context of childbirth. Unpublished manuscript. University of Rhode Island, Kingston, RI.

Hogue, C. (1985). Social support. In J. Hall & B. Weaver (Eds.), *Distributive nursing practice: A systems approach to community health* (2nd ed.) (pp. 58–81). Philadelphia: J.B. Lippincott.

Janicki, J. (1981). Anguish: A concept analysis. Unpublished manuscript. University of Rhode Island, Kingston, RI.

Kaplan, A. (1964). *The conduct of inquiry: Methodology for behavioral science.* New York: Chandler.

Keith, J. (1988). Participant observation. In K. Schaie, R. Campbell, W. Meredith, & S. Rawlings (Eds.), *Methodological issues in aging research* (pp. 211–230). New York: Springer.

Kim, H. S. (1983). *The nature of theoretical thinking in nursing.* Norwalk, Conn: Appleton-Century-Crofts.

Leininger, M. M. (1985). Ethnography and ethnonursing: Models and modes of qualitative data analysis. In M. M. Leininger (Ed.), *Qualitative research methods in nursing* (pp. 33–71). New York: Grune & Stratton.

Lofland, J. (1976). *Doing social life.* New York: John Wiley & Sons.

Lofland, J., & Lofland, L. H. (1984). *Analyzing social settings: A guide to qualitative observation and analysis.* Belmont, Calif: Wadsworth.

McCall, G. J., & Simmons, J. L. (1969). *Issues in participant observation: A text and reader.* Reading, Mass: Addison-Wesley.

May, R. (1972). The nature of creativity. In H. H. Anderson (Ed.), *Interdisciplinary symposia on creativity* (pp. 55–68). New York: Harper & Row.

Meleis, A. I. (1985). *Theoretical nursing: Development and progress.* Philadelphia: JB Lippincott.

Messerschmidt, D. A. (1981). *Anthropologists at home in North America: Methods and issues in the study of one's own society.* New York: Cambridge University Press.

Miles, M. B., & Huberman, A. M. (1984). *Qualitative data analysis.* Beverly Hills: Sage.

Nagel, E. (1961). *The structure of science.* New York: Harcourt, Brace & World.

National League for Nursing. (1972). *Criteria for the appraisal of baccalaureate and higher degree programs in nursing.* New York: The League.

Norris, C. M. (1982). *Concept clarification in nursing.* Rockville, Md: Aspen.

Panzarine, S. (1985). Coping: Conceptual and methodological issues. *Advances in Nursing Science, 7*(4), 49–58.

Pelto, P. J. (1970). *Anthropological research: The structure of inquiry.* New York: Cambridge University.

Pelto, P. J., & Pelto, G. H. (1984). *Anthropologist research: The structure of inquiry* (2nd ed.). New York: Cambridge University.

Reed, P. G., & Leonard, V. E. (1990). An analysis of the concept of self-neglect. *Advances in Nursing Science, 12*(1), 39–53.

Reilly, H. A. (1982). A concept analysis of creativity. Unpublished manuscript. University of Rhode Island, Kingston, RI.

Rew, L., & Barrow, E. M. (1987). Intuition: A neglected hallmark of nursing knowledge. *Advances in Nursing Science, 10*(1), 49–62.

Reynolds, P. D. (1971). *A primer in theory construction.* New York: Bobbs-Merrill.

Roberts, N. (1982). An analysis of the concept of empathy. Unpublished manuscript. University of Rhode Island, Kingston, RI.

Rogers, R. (1972). Toward a theory of creativity. In H. H. Anderson (Ed.), *Interdisciplinary symposia on creativity* (pp. 69–82). New York: Harper & Row.

St. Angelo L. (1983). The concept of bonding. Unpublished manuscript. University of Rhode Island, Kingston, RI.

Sartori, G. (1984). *Social science concepts: A systematic analysis.* Beverly Hills: Sage.

Schatzman, L., & Strauss, A. L. (1973). *Field research: Strategies for a natural sociology.* Englewood Cliffs, NJ: Prentice-Hall.

Schwartz-Barcott, D. (1986). Conceptualization: Concept formation. In N. Wells & C. Bridges (Eds.), *Strategies for theory development in nursing III.* Proceedings of the Third Annual Nursing Science Colloquium. Boston University, Boston, April, 1986, pp. 19–35.

Schwartz-Barcott, D., & Kim, H. S. (1986). A hybrid model for concept development. In P. L. Chinn (Ed.), *Nursing research methodology: Issues and implementations.* Rockville, Md: Aspen.

Seidler, S. (1984). Fear in the patient undergoing a coronary artery bypass graft. Unpublished manuscript. University of Rhode Island, Kingston, RI.

Spradley, J. P. (1980). *Participant observation.* New York: Holt, Rinehart and Winston.

Strauss, A. L. (1987). *Qualitative analysis for social scientists.* New York: Cambridge University Press.

Sundeen, S. J., Stuart, G. W., Rankin, E.A. & Cohen, S. A. (1976). *Nurse-client interaction: Implementing the nursing process.* St Louis: Mosby.

Taylor, S. J., & Bogdan, R. (1984). *Introduction to qualitative research methods: The search for meanings* (2nd ed.). New York: John Wiley & Sons.

Testa, G. (1980). A participant observation study of the concept of psycho-social withdrawal in the aged nursing home resident. Unpublished manuscript. University of Rhode Island, Kingston, RI.

Van Maanen, J. (1988). *Tales of the field: On writing ethnography.* Chicago: University of Chicago Press.

Walker, L. O., & Avant, K. C. (1988). *Strategies for theory construction in nursing.* Norwalk, Conn: Appleton & Lange.

Wax, R. H. (1986). *Doing fieldwork: Warnings and advice.* Chicago: University of Chicago Press.

Werner, O., & Schoepfle, G. M. (1987). *Foundations of ethnography and interviewing* (Vol. 1). Beverly Hills: Sage.

Whyte, W. F. (1984). *Learning from the field: A guide from experience.* Beverly Hills: Sage.

Wilson, H. S. (1982). *Deinstitutionalized residential approaches for the severely and mentally disordered patient: The soteria house approach.* New York: Grune & Stratton.

Wilson, H. S. (1986). Presencing—social control of schizophrenics in an antipsychiatric community: Doing grounded theory. In P. Munhall & C. Oiler (Eds.), *Nursing research: A qualitative perspective* (pp. 131–144). Norwalk, Conn: Appleton-Century-Crofts.

Wilson, J. (1969). *Thinking with concepts.* London: Cambridge University Press.

Zola, I. K. (1983). *Socio-medical inquiries: Recollections, reflections and reconsiderations.* Philadelphia: Temple University Press.

Chapter 9

A Concept Analysis of Withdrawal: Application of the Hybrid Model of Concept Development

GERALDINE VERHULST AND DONNA SCHWARTZ-BARCOTT

*W*ithdrawal is a highly pervasive, yet relatively underdeveloped concept in nursing. In the nursing literature, withdrawal has been used to characterize the behavior of the mentally ill patient, the behavioral responses of patients to acute and chronic physical illness, as well as the responses of nurses to situations of anxiety and stress (Beland, 1980; Davis, 1975; Friedrick & Lively, 1981; Hutchinson, 1987; Jacobson, 1983; Jasmin & Trygstad, 1979; Kramer, 1974; Peplau, 1963; Schmidt, 1981; Scully, 1980; Tudor, 1952). Yet, any attempt at greater understanding of withdrawal is hindered by its lack of explication and development in nursing. The term is not even cited as a subject in the *Cumulative Index to Nursing and Allied Health Literature.* When it is used, it is often embedded in other phenomena, such as protective isolationism (Kramer, 1974), distancing (Beland, 1980; Jacobson, 1983; Scully, 1980), psychological immobilization (Friedrick & Lively, 1981), panic (Oden, 1963), anxiety (Peplau, 1963) and depression (Jasmin & Trygstad, 1979). Most recently, withdrawal is being used in the nursing diagnosis literature as a defining characteristic for the diagnoses of fear, pain, social isolation, and spiritual distress (Kim, McFarland, & McLane, 1987).

It is this elusive quality of withdrawal that led us to question its underlying meaning. The following concept analysis was undertaken to establish a base for further theoretical and empirical understanding of this phenomenon in nursing. The following are the specific questions addressed: To what extent is there a universal meaning and definition of withdrawal? Have there been any attempts at measuring withdrawal? If so, to what extent are these measurements linked with existing definitions? To what extent can any of these definitions or measurements be applied, and if not, what refinements are needed?

This chapter is an attempt to answer these questions by using the hybrid model of concept development (Schwartz-Barcott & Kim, chapter 8) to further define and measure withdrawal. The subsequent theoretical phase gives a review of behavioral, social science, and nursing literature where the concept has been partially defined and used with varying degrees of frequency. The aim is to present a broad cross-disciplinary approach focusing first on existing definitions and second on measurements of withdrawal. This literature review, which was begun in phase one and extended in phase two of the hybrid model, is then used as a basis for comparison and integration with empirical observations of withdrawal among nursing home residents.* Finally, a refined definition and operationalization of withdrawal is proposed based on this theoretical and empirical analysis.

Theoretical Phase

DEFINING WITHDRAWAL

In its simplest form, withdrawal can be conceived as an instinctive defensive mechanism of lower animals characterized by physical retreat to escape from danger (Edmunds, 1974). In a more complex form, withdrawal has been conceptualized in the field of psychiatry as an unconscious, intrapsychic process indicating a retreat from objective reality (Ziegler, 1933). Withdrawal, as a form of retreat, was initially described by Bleuler (1912) in the *Theory of Schizophrenic Negativism* as the "autistic withdrawing of the patient into his phantasies" (p.2). Historically, the early work of Bleuler (1912) and Kraepelin (1904) led to negative symptoms as forming the conceptual core of schizophrenia (Andreasen & Flaum, 1991) with blunted affect, emotional withdrawal, and motor retardation as the items most frequently identified (deLeon, Wilson, & Simpson, 1989). King (1956) operationalized withdrawal as a dimension in schizophrenia defining environmental withdrawal, or withdrawal from reality, as behavior directed away from at least two types of stimuli, people and things. Furthermore, Frieswyk (1977) expanded the notion of fantasy in withdrawal suggesting that "fantasy withdrawal" is the degree to which a person is withdrawn into self-absorption of thoughts, fantasies, wishes, and somatic experiences to the exclusion of reality. Drawing on these earlier ideas about schizophrenia, Schmidt (1981) provided a broader meaning to withdrawal by defining the concept as:

> *a behavioral pattern characterized by an individual's retreat from interpersonal relationships and contacts with the external environ-*

*This concept analysis and fieldwork was initially undertaken by Geraldine (Testa) Verhulst in the early 1980s as part of her master's level course work. This chapter expands on these endeavors, including an update of the literature, and was written in collaboration with Donna Schwartz-Barcott.

ment... a reduced response to external stimuli and increased response to internal stimuli... withdrawal may be manifested in a wide variety of behaviors ranging from mild to severe based upon the individual's degree of personality disintegration. (p.28)

Withdrawal as a personality trait was supported by Pallister (1933) who likened the negative or withdrawal attitude to the concept of introversion. Weinstein, Kahn, and Slote (1956) found through premorbid personality assessments that withdrawal, silence, and avoidance were patients' habitual modes of adaptation to stressful situations. Premorbid personality disorders, such as schizotypal have emphasized social withdrawal as a major aspect of the schizoid temperament (Kendler, 1985). Additionally, childhood temperament studies (Thomas & Chess, 1977) have incorporated approach or withdrawal behavior as one of the nine categories used in defining temperament characteristics.

Withdrawal as a negative phenomenon has also been explicated in the early child psychiatry literature. The work of Spitz and Wolf (1946) provided highly poignant descriptions of withdrawal in infants under extreme situations of stress. During an 18-month period of observation, they described a syndrome called anaclitic depression in 19 of the 123 institutionalized infants. This syndrome was characterized by a progressive and profound withdrawal of the infants from their environment. In the following example, Spitz and Wolf (1946) described the sudden withdrawal of a once friendly seven-month-old girl. The child began to show signs of apprehensiveness. Over the next two weeks, these signs became accentuated and were accompanied by frequent crying. By four weeks,

she could no longer be approached. No amount of persuasion helped. Whenever approached she sat up and wailed. Two weeks later, she would lie on her face, indifferent to the outside world, not interested in other children living in the same room. Only strong stimulation could get her out of her apathy. She would sit up and stare at the observer wide-eyed, a tragic expression in her face, silent. She would not accept toys, in fact she withdrew from them into the farthest corner of her bed. (p. 315)

Furthermore, Engel and Reichsman (1956) observed a striking behavioral pattern defined as a depression-withdrawal reaction over a nine-month period in the hospitalized infant Monica. This reaction typically occurred when the infant was confronted alone by a stranger and was characterized by muscular inactivity, hypotonia, a sad facial expression, decreased gastric secretion, and eventually a sleep state.

Most recently the child psychology literature has examined the problem of social withdrawal in noninstitutionalized school aged children. Social withdrawal or isolation has been increasingly recognized as a serious behavioral disorder with implications for maladjustment in later life (Ballard, 1983; Greenwood, Walker, & Haps, 1977). Internalizing/withdrawal and externalizing/aggression have been identified as two fundamental dimensions of childhood maladjustment in which psychological problems can be classified (Achenbach & Edelbrock, 1978). Greenwood and others (1977) suggested that the concept of social withdrawal implies avoidance of social contacts and low rates of peer interaction, together with relatively high rates of other behaviors such as self-play, hovering, and observation of others.

Other descriptors of the withdrawn child have included shy, submissive, sad, fearful, and easy to offend. Ollendick, Oswald, and Francis (1989) found that withdrawn children, as compared to popular children, interacted less frequently with peers, engaged in more solitary play, and were often observed to be alone.

A variety of terms, usually negative in connotation, such as apathy reaction and withdrawal, have been used to describe the psychosocial effects of institutionalization in the aged (Lieberman, Prock, & Tobin, 1968). Relocation, particularly institutionalization, has been considered a stressful event (Borup, 1983), with the most severe stress lasting through the initial adjustment period of two months (Tobin & Lieberman, 1976). Chenitz (1983) showed that the negative response of "resigned resistance" emerged in this adjustment period and was characterized by a range of behaviors including withdrawal. Gurland, Dean, and Cross (1983) suggested that withdrawal in the aged is not an isolated symptom, but is often seen in depression and may be accompanied by loneliness and loss of self-esteem. Moses (1985) defined withdrawn nursing home residents as those who showed little emotional response to nursing care and who could not be reached by existing activities.

In contrast to these impressions, the notion of withdrawal as an adaptive process indicating successful adjustment to aging emerged as a central theme in the disengagement theory. Disengagement as perceived by Cumming and Henry (1961) is a mutually satisfying process of withdrawal between the aged person and society. However, with the emergence of other psychosocial theories of aging, disengagement has been challenged as a desirable process of aging (Brehm, 1968; Burbank, 1986; Maddox, 1965).

Other social scientists have viewed withdrawal as a transient coping mechanism illuminating its positive adaptive function. Hamburg, Hamburg, and deGoza (1953) explored patients' emotional recovery from life-threatening burns and found that withdrawal was used as a coping mechanism during the first few weeks following injury. Sapirstein (1948) had emphasized this idea earlier, suggesting that the temporary use of withdrawal can be useful as a transitory state for energy conservation. Ironside (1980) depicted "conservation-withdrawal" as a universal feature of survivor behavior defined as "a biological threshold mechanism whereby survival of the organism is supported by processes of disengagement in activity from the external environment" (p. 163). The purpose of conservation-withdrawal is to assist the person, both physically and psychologically, in preparation for "action-engagement" in order to meet environmental and situational demands.

The nursing literature has further empirical evidence of withdrawal as a purposeful coping strategy used temporarily in situations of stress. Cochrane (1983) studied social withdrawal experiences of healthy adults defining the concept as "physical or psychological movement from other people and into oneself" (p. 23). Three types of withdrawal were identified: active, reactive, and passive; active withdrawal was reported as a transient coping mechanism and was viewed as a time to clarify thoughts and prepare for action. The potential for a progressive maladaptive form of passive withdrawal was also supported.

Withdrawal has also been discussed as a *nursing* strategy to handle anxiety associated with clinical nursing problems (Hurteau, 1963). Kramer (1974) viewed withdrawing as a form of "protective isolationism," a strategy used to cope with stressful work environments. These strategies could be seen in the new graduate nurses' withdrawal to bed, sleeping more hours than usual, and withdrawal to the night shift. Similarly, Hutchinson (1987) found withdrawal to be a self-care strategy used by nurses to cope with job stress. Self-reports from hospital nurses indicated that withdrawal increased their emotional control protecting them from chronic emotional drain. Withdrawal behaviors were described as both physical and emotional, in which physical withdrawal helped the nurse to withdraw emotionally. Examples of withdrawal behaviors by nurses are leaving the unit, working the night shift, taking time out by eating alone, and ultimately resigning as an extreme form of withdrawal in a hopeless situation.

Withdrawal as a *patient's* control strategy over nurses was presented by Glaser and Strauss (1965) in their trajectories of dying patients. They suggested that withdrawal is the patient's most extreme control over the pace of interaction with nurses. Furthermore, this type of withdrawal is more than giving up. It is an implicit message that the patient is finished with everything and everyone, including the nursing staff (p. 89).

In a classic study of withdrawal, Tudor (1952) demonstrated that withdrawal can be used by both the *nurse* and *patient.* Tudor identified the problem of mutual withdrawal between the nursing staff and schizophrenic patients. She argued that the nurses' social interaction pattern of avoidance reinforced the patients' withdrawal and was the dominant reason for the maintenance of the patients' mental illness.

In summary, the literature reviewed here illuminates the diverse use of withdrawal in behavioral, social, and nursing science. It has been used to characterize animal defensive behavior, mental health and social problems, personality traits, human responses to stress ranging from severe deprivation to the more usual stresses of daily life, and as an active coping strategy. Additionally, withdrawal has been described as both an adaptive and maladaptive coping mechanism that at times may be progressive.

Yet, explicit definitions of withdrawal were seldom encountered. There was, implicitly, a moderate degree of agreement in the shared impressions and terms (e.g., retreat, avoidance, disengagement, autism, and isolation) used to express the idea of withdrawal. Most fundamentally, withdrawal seemed to entail some form of retreat. Earlier definitions referred to a physical action—a moving out of the immediate environment. Later, this physical action was associated with emotional inaction, rather than actual physical removal from the setting. Recently, the focus has been on retreat from social interaction. Thus, it appears that withdrawal includes three major dimensions: physical, emotional, and social.

Finally, there is a paucity of literature about withdrawal as a separate phenomenon. There is a need to distinguish the behavioral and conceptual features of withdrawal from other closely related concepts such as avoidance, depression, and social isolation. In the process of defining withdrawal, it is important to define what is not withdrawal.

MEASURING WITHDRAWAL

Researchers have attempted to assess the physical, social, and emotional dimensions of withdrawal, yet the application of specific measures has been dependent upon the researcher's point of focus and conceptualization of withdrawal. Consequently, the measurement of withdrawal, like its definition, has been partially developed with a diverse range of measures. Of those encountered, the majority have focused on social withdrawal.

The three most common methods of identifying socially withdrawn children and measuring interactive behavior have been based upon sociometric peer rating measures, behavioral observational measures of social interaction frequency or duration, and teacher nominations or ratings (Greenwood et al., 1977).

Researchers examining social withdrawal in adult subjects have used self-reported measures of withdrawal such as a reduction in social participation (Lowenthal & Boler, 1965) and accounts of mental visualization techniques to re-experience situations of social withdrawal (Cochrane, 1983). Similarly, Hutchinson (1987) used nurses' self-reported measures of coping mechanisms and found that withdrawal was used as an active coping behavior. A frequently reported social indicator was that of needing to be alone.

Measurement of the emotional dimension in withdrawal as a reduced affective response has been assessed by projective techniques such as Rorschach responses (Frieswyk, 1977) and Hand Test Withdrawal Responses (Wagner, 1978). Daum (1983) used projective drawings of human stick figures to measure emotional indicators of withdrawal in delinquent adolescent boys. Drawings characterized by the absence of facial features, omitted arms, profile views, and dim facial features were indicative of withdrawal.

Nonspecific rating scales such as the Brief Psychiatric Rating Scale (Overall & Gorham, 1962) have been used to measure the construct of negative symptoms in schizophrenia with emotional withdrawal as one of a 16-symptom construct on a seven-point scale to quickly assess the degree of pathology in psychiatric patients. Emotional withdrawal has been determined by the feeling of the interviewers that an "invisible barrier" existed between themselves and the patients. Facial expressions, voice quality, and expressive movements have entered into the evaluation process.

Attitudinal measurement of withdrawal was done by Pallister (1933) through an adjustment questionnaire using a semantic differential scale based on approach or avoidance responses to social situations. More recently, the concept of psychological readiness for withdrawal, perceived as a predisposition towards passivity, solitude, inactivity, and reduced emotional intensity, was used as an attitudinal measure of disengagement potential assessed on a Guttman Scale of Disengagement (Tissue, 1968). Furthermore, McDonnell and Beck (1986) reported that childhood temperament studies have used the category of approach or withdrawal to new stimuli—be it to a new person, food, or toy—in operationalizing the concept of temperament in which approach responses are positive and withdrawal reactions are negative whether displayed by measure of mood expression (i.e., crying, fussing, grimacing) or measures of motor activity (i.e., moving away, spitting out new food, or pushing away a new toy).

In contrast to the previous measures that focused on a specific dimension of withdrawal, Schmidt (1981) compiled a list of 24 behavioral indicators along four categories: physical, verbal, affective, and disruption in reality as a measure for sample selection of withdrawn schizophrenic subjects. Indicators were developed from descriptions in psychiatric nursing literature. Neither the indicators nor categories were weighted; the presence of five or more indicators constituted withdrawal.

Measurement of physical withdrawal was not dealt with as a separate dimension; yet in many descriptive studies physical characteristics were a frequent inference of withdrawal from self-reported data and behavioral observations (Engel & Reichsman, 1956; Fields, 1985; Hutchinson, 1987; Ironside, 1980; Leyn, 1972; Moses, 1985; Schmidt, 1981; Spitz & Wolf, 1946; Tudor, 1952; Weinstein et al., 1956). Empirical observations emerged from these studies that further support conceptualizing withdrawal along the three dimensions of physical, social, and emotional generating indicators, which may add empirical relevance to the measurement of withdrawal. Drawing on the efforts of Schmidt (1981), we developed a list of behavioral indicators of withdrawal, in terms of its physical, social, and emotional dimensions (see Table 9–1).

This table was derived by analyzing the concept of withdrawal into its

Table 9–1   *Indicators of Withdrawal*

Physical

Retreat (i.e., to bed, corners, closets, and lockers, under covers, and movement away from people) Staying in room	Spitz & Wolf, 1946; Tudor, 1952; King, 1956; O'Connor, 1969; Leyn, 1972; Kramer, 1974; Thomas & Chess, 1977; Schmidt, 1981
Protective posturing (i.e., averted face, turning away, shrinking position, flexing of knees to abdomen)	Spitz & Wolf, 1946; Engel & Reichsman, 1956; Tudor, 1952
Diminished movement Immobile	Spitz & Wolf, 1946; Engel & Reichsman, 1956; Weinstein et al., 1956; Ironside, 1980; Hutchinson, 1987
Repetitive rhythmic movement	Weinstein et al., 1956; Fields, 1985; Moses, 1985
Prolonged sleep Wandering	Engel & Reichsman, 1956; Weinstein et al., 1956; Kramer, 1974; Ironside, 1980; Ziegler, 1933; Ollendick et al., 1989

Social

Avoidance of people Low social interaction	Tudor, 1952; King, 1956; Leyn, 1972; O'Connor, 1969; Schmidt, 1981; Ollendick et al., 1989
Alone	King, 1956; Fields, 1985; Hutchinson, 1987; Serbin et al., 1987; Ollendick et al., 1989
Shy	Ross et al., 1965; O'Connor, 1969; Ollendick et al., 1989
Solitary play	Ollendick et al., 1989
Meditative silence	Ironside, 1980; Spitz & Wolf, 1946
Silence	Tudor, 1952; Fields, 1985; Moses, 1985
Slow verbal response Nonsensical speech Monotone voice	Weinstein et al., 1956; Schmidt, 1981; Moses, 1985
Missing scheduled appointments	Fields, 1985

Emotional

Blank facial expression Frozen, rigid facial expression. Sad facial expression (i.e., face sagged, furrowed brow, corners of mouth turned down)	Spitz & Wolf, 1946; Engel & Reichsman, 1956; Moses, 1985

Table 9–1	*Indicators of Withdrawal* Continued
Emotional cont'd	
Closed eyes	Engel & Reichsman, 1956; Weinstein et al., 1956
Wide eyed	Spitz & Wolf, 1946; Schmidt, 1981
Staring into space	Spitz & Wolf, 1946; Tudor, 1952; Weinstein et al., 1956; Ollendick et al., 1989
Aloofness	Leyn, 1972; Schmidt, 1981
Inattention	Tudor, 1952; Weinstein et al., 1956
Detachment "no nothing feeling"	Ironside, 1980; Cochrane, 1983
Confusion	Moses, 1985
Apathy	Spitz & Wolf, 1946; Schmidt, 1981
Delusions/hallucinations	Schmidt, 1981

various behavioral dimensions that can be observed directly, and therefore evaluated more reliably than those based on inference and self-reported data. The choice of indicators was guided by two major considerations. First, several of the items were drawn from measures used in studies on social withdrawal, thus tapping behavioral characteristics already demonstrated to be reliably identifiable. Second, items were selected that were empirically derived through descriptive studies in the literature review. It should be noted that verbal indicators have been included in the social dimension and facial expressive cues within the emotional dimension of withdrawal.

It is apparent from reviewing Table 9–1 that a number of measurement problems exist. First, and most importantly, is the need to determine construct validity of the dimensions used to operationalize withdrawal. Second is the need to determine interrater reliability of the items used as indicators within each dimension. Third, because this might be a limited pool of the items that represent the empirical reality of withdrawal, further descriptive studies need to be conducted to validate indicators, add to this pool, and ultimately discern the importance of any one indicator over another. Furthermore, even though an observational approach is used for the measurement of withdrawal, there are several indicators in the emotional dimension that seem refractory to empirical study. Therefore, their assessment must rely on less precise measures such as the projective techniques and self-report measures.

Following these endeavors, an instrument to measure withdrawal could be developed drawing from the most reliable items. Measurement of this concept beyond the nominal level, by rank-ordering the indicators on the basis of frequency or severity, would be crucial in determining the progression of withdrawal while advancing knowledge in nursing science.

The Fieldwork Phase

SETTING THE STAGE

Shortly after the literature review was initiated, a fieldwork phase was begun to examine withdrawal among nursing home residents. This population was selected for several reasons. Earlier experiences by the authors and colleagues suggested that withdrawal had been encountered rather frequently in this population. In the initial literature review, withdrawal had been explicitly linked with the aged. Additionally, it was anticipated that withdrawal would be highly frequent in the context of relocation and the stress associated with adjustment. Lastly, the nursing home setting was a feasible, practical, and not overly familiar environment in which one of the authors (Verhulst) would undertake a three-month period of participant observation.

Based on a beginning exploration of the literature, the following working definition was used to start this study. Withdrawal is a behavioral response of retreat from the external environment that may be progressive and manifested by a variety of behaviors. This definition was reconceptualized several times as the literature review continued and, as will be evident in the final analytical phase, refined on the basis of this fieldwork. Additionally, several questions guided this fieldwork phase. These questions stemmed from the focus on definition and measurement found in the hybrid model of concept development (Schwartz-Barcott & Kim, chapter 8) and from the initial exploration of the literature on withdrawal.

1. Is there evidence of the existence of withdrawal among nursing home residents?
2. If so, to what extent do existing definitions sufficiently capture the essential nature of this phenomenon?
3. What indicators best reflect the existence of withdrawal?
4. Is there any evidence of withdrawal becoming progressive?
5. If so, under what conditions does withdrawal become progressive?

To obtain a rich and full understanding of withdrawal, investigation was done through overt participant observation using unstructured observational techniques during situational and casual conversation, with incidental questioning, as forms of informal interviewing. The focus of observations centered on four residents, each of whom the researcher saw for one hour a week over a three-month period. Other sources of data included medical records and interviews with nursing staff, social workers, and activity directors. Journals and field notes were organized according to Schatzman and Strauss's (1973) notation system of observational, theoretical, and methodological notes.

Although the basic questions did not alter over time, observations surfaced that changed this researcher's earlier perceptions of withdrawal. The researcher believed at the start of the literature review and before gathering field observations that people need social activity to facilitate adaptation to a nursing home and that withdrawal is negative in that it inhibits the meeting of these social needs. During fieldwork, these beliefs were called into question, as will be discussed later in the analysis.

NEGOTIATING ENTRY

The researcher had no prior affiliation with the research settings, which were accredited multilevel nursing homes located in Rhode Island. Permission to conduct the study was granted by the administrators, and residents verbally consented to be interviewed. Participation or nonparticipation in the study had no effect on residents' care, position in the nursing home, nor posed any risk of harm. The term *withdrawal* was purposely not mentioned, yet residents were aware that the researcher was a graduate nursing student collecting information on peoples' thoughts and feelings about living in a nursing home.

SELECTING CASES

The rationale for selecting cases was oriented toward further development and refinement of the concept of withdrawal. Therefore, the researcher selected residents who exhibited withdrawal as determined through nomination by the nursing staff and by meeting the criteria of three indicators, selected from measures used in the literature, which the researcher believed best represented the physical, emotional, and social dimensions of withdrawal. These indicators were: (1) spending the majority of the time alone and physically removed from other residents, (2) rarely, if ever, interacting with other residents or participating in social activities within the nursing home, and (3) exhibiting a detached, aloof, indifferent or apathetic attitude toward others. An additional goal of the researcher was to examine the idea that withdrawal is progressive. Consequently, residents were selected who had been in the nursing home for varying lengths of time. One resident who was newly relocated to the nursing home was selected for the purpose of examining withdrawal from an adjustment perspective.

Although the residents nominated by the nursing staff met the listed criteria, it was evident that several of them were experiencing conditions of immobility (bedridden), senility, dying from terminal illness, depression or side effects from psychotropic medications. Because withdrawal might be difficult to distinguish from these previously mentioned conditions, restrictions were placed on the selection of residents to increase the probability of encountering withdrawal. Thus, residents were omitted if they had physical or emotional disorders such as deafness, blindness, senility, aphasia, terminal diseases, or psychiatric disorders that might have overwhelmingly contributed to withdrawal behavior. Residents also were omitted who had been receiving medications that had side effects that could alter a person's emotional response. Finally, residents needed to be able to speak and understand the English language, be oriented to person, but not necessarily place and time, yet not be in a continuous confusional state.

The actual selection of four residents (three men and one woman) took two weeks from the time of negotiating entry. The three male residents were representative of the overall nursing home population being of Canadian origin and formerly working as laborers. The one female resident selected was not typical of the nursing home population because she was of Italian descent and had been raised in a middle-class home.

In addition to the key questions used to guide this inquiry, residents were asked to talk about their lives (e.g., family, friends, activities) before they entered the nursing home. The purpose of these inquiries was to gain a greater sense of the psychosocial context in which withdrawal was being observed. Additionally, they were asked many questions about how life was different for them now. Specifically, they were asked to discuss feelings of loneliness and depression because these concepts had been identified in the literature as being associated with the aged and withdrawal.

PRESENTATION OF CASES

The cases that follow are presented in relation to three residents, referred to by the pseudonyms of Mrs. Bianco, Mr. Charpentier, and Mr. DuBois. Although the fieldwork examined withdrawal in four cases, only three will be presented because the withdrawal encountered was highly similar in two residents. The framework for case presentation begins with a brief description of withdrawal by the nursing staff, followed by the resident's perception of the psychosocial context leading to relocation, and ending with the researcher's observations. Next is a primary analysis of withdrawal focusing on meaning and measurement of the concept. Concluding the case presentations, a final analytical phase is presented in which withdrawal is compared and contrasted across cases including a comparison of the findings with the literature. The working definition of withdrawal is refined based on the fieldwork findings. The chapter ends with ideas for future investigations and addresses the usefulness of the hybrid model of concept development as a method for the concept analysis of withdrawal.

Case 1: Mrs. Bianco. Mrs. Bianco is a 65-year-old widow of Italian descent who has been in the nursing home for one year. The nursing staff refers to her as "withdrawn, difficult, and moody." Nursing notes reflect that she stays in her room with the door closed, never talks to other residents, and refuses to participate in social activities. She has a private room and spends most of her time alone. The staff relates that she is very resistant to their attempts to get her socially involved with other residents. Her behavior annoys the nursing staff who commented among themselves that Mrs. Bianco acts as though "she is superior to the other residents."

Mrs. Bianco relates that she is a college educated woman who never worked outside of the home because she spent the majority of her adult life caring for her aging parents. After her parents' deaths, she married and spent her time caring for her home and developing an interest in oil painting. She describes herself as a cultured woman who appreciates good art, music, food, and wine.

Four months before she entered the nursing home, Mrs. Bianco's husband died suddenly of a heart attack. She describes her reaction as "panic, shock, and total grief." "After my husband's death, no one cared about me. We really didn't have any close friends or family." The only family members are Mrs. Bianco's brother and sister who, she recalls, rarely visited after the funeral. She describes her relationships with her siblings as "full of strife since childhood."

Mrs. Bianco saw no purpose to life and a pattern of daily drinking developed. She could not recall much toward the end, but eventually was hospitalized for treatment of malnutrition and weakness. It seems that Mrs. Bianco stopped answering the telephone, which precipitated a visit by her brother. He found her to be stuporous, thin, and untidy. "He must have called an ambulance and had me brought to the hospital, I really don't remember." The medical record reflects that she was treated for alcoholism and malnutrition.

She spoke of resenting her brother who took advantage of her weakened condition by "taking control of everything." It seems that he gained control of her estate and arranged to have Mrs. Bianco transferred from the hospital to a nursing home for the purpose of gaining physical strength. "I feel like a victim, everything taken away from me and brought to a place like this." She maintains weekly contact with her brother, relating that he is her "only link to the outside world." Mrs. Bianco resents being called an alcoholic and particularly the nursing staffs' unsuccessful attempt to have her attend weekly Alcoholic Anonymous meetings. She does admit to drinking out of control, yet attributes this behavior to despair over her husband's death. "I just didn't care anymore." Mrs. Bianco does maintain some hope for the future, particularly since she has been feeling physically stronger. Her goal is to convince her brother to allow her to leave the nursing home.

The only time Mrs. Bianco leaves her room is to smoke cigarettes. She often spoke of the lack of privacy. Even in a private room, nurses would enter without knocking. She also believed some staff were taking her personal items and had locks placed on her closet to prevent this theft. Mrs. Bianco feels that the activities within the nursing home are not interesting, nor does she intend to mix with the other residents in such "silly things" as bingo and cards. Recently, a volunteer art instructor began teaching weekly classes. Mrs. Bianco has started to attend these classes and to learning to do charcoal sketches. I observed her at several of the classes and noticed that the only person she spoke with was the teacher. She sat at a table by herself away from the other residents. On one occasion, I accompanied her back to her room and had the opportunity to note her response to other residents. As we passed the lounge areas and residents' room she would look straight ahead as if she was ignoring the existence of these people.

Mrs. Bianco would remain aloof and displayed little facial expression when talking. She would physically distance herself from the reseacher and would rarely make eye contact. Usually she would place restrictions on the time and length of conversations. She met with the researcher in her room and was quite candid saying, "I would not even talk with you if I did not like the way you looked or acted." She denied feeling lonely, yet related that she was a little depressed. Depression seemed to be improving because she slept less often during the daytime and participated in the art classes. Often she would reminisce about her marriage and fond memories of her husband. Toward the end of this study, she shared with the researcher the charcoal sketches she had done in the art class. Although her future was one big "question mark," she maintained hope that things would change and she would someday leave the nursing home.

Certainly, Mrs. Bianco's behavior gives an overall impression of withdrawal reflecting some aspects of all three dimensions identified in the literature. The physical dimension is evident by her retreat to her room and her physically distancing herself from other residents, including the researcher. The emotional indicators include her expressionless face, aloofness, and attitudinal behavior of ignoring the presence of other residents, whereas social withdrawal is apparent by her avoidance of social interaction and being alone.

Withdrawal emerged as an active, purposeful behavior with no evidence of progression during the year of nursing home residence. For Mrs. Bianco, withdrawal is essentially a strategic maneuver to protect herself from the inherent stress of an environment that is incongruent with her self-concept. Factors that seemed to influence the development of withdrawal are the recent loss of a significant other with subsequent depression, minimal social support, loss of control (no input into the decision concerning her relocation), and a change in lifestyle imposed by the nursing home.

Case 2: Mr. Charpentier. Mr. Charpentier is a 90-year-old widower of French Canadian descent who has been in the nursing home for three years. The nursing staff describes him as "withdrawn, sits alone all day, refuses to participate in social activities, silent, occasionally uses foul language, forgetful and sometimes confused."

A hip fracture resulting from a fall led to hospitalization, with subsequent relocation to the nursing home. Before this fall, he had been living alone in an apartment managing for himself. His only daughter maintains little contact with him. His former occupation is listed as self-employed brick-layer.

During the initial encounter the researcher found Mr. Charpentier sitting in a chair in the corner of his room. He did not notice her presence, appeared preoccupied, and was twiddling his thumbs in a repetitious motion while quietly talking to himself. Each week the researcher found him in the same chair, in the same corner, performing the same hand motion, and talking to himself. Initially this self-dialogue seemed nonsensical, but careful listening disclosed that he was carrying on a conversation with someone. For the first several weeks, this behavior continued as the researcher sat quietly by his side.

Establishing a baseline mental status at the time of relocation seemed crucial in understanding Mr. Charpentier's withdrawal. Investigation revealed that he was "alert, oriented with a quiet affect." Cognitive and intellectual deficits were minimal. There was some disagreement among the nursing staff as to Mr. Charpentier's current mental status. Several believed he was confused, while others disagreed suggesting that he was pretending to be confused so that people would not bother him or talk with him. Several nursing assistants related that he would talk to them on occasion. They found his behavior frustrating, particularly because he could talk and walk, but he just "doesn't bother to anymore."

The researcher continued with weekly visits, sitting next to him, touching his hand, and repeating his name. After three weeks, he stopped the repetitious hand movements and began talking. He rambled on about people in the past, foods he used to cook, and things he did. It was difficult to informally interview Mr. Charpentier because his flow of reminiscing would be interrupted only with periods of silence. On the few occasions in which the researcher was able to focus the conversation on the nursing home environment and his feelings toward life now, he responded that such talk was a waste of time because "life is useless now, nothing to do and nowhere to go." Once he said, "the only way I will ever leave here is in a coffin." He spoke negatively of his daughter, relating that she "didn't care and had no time for him."

In subsequent encounters, the researcher found Mr. Charpentier to be alert, oriented, and willing to talk. Most of his conversation was about the past. He denied feeling lonely or depressed, but was waiting his time out until the "good lord takes me." Often, upon entering his room, the researcher found him twiddling his thumbs, talking quietly to himself. Yet this behavior would stop when he began talking. He became upset and swore if anyone tried to rearrange his room. For example, the chair was placed in the far corner away from the window. Once the researcher suggested that it could be turned toward the window for a better view. He commented, "why bother, I've seen everything there is to in life." He referred to his corner as "my world now." He also became upset if his roommate's belongings were placed on his side of the room. He purposefully avoided his roommate calling him "a foolish old man." Occasionally, if other residents were not in the halls, he would take short walks with the researcher. He often peered into the residents' rooms making derogatory comments such as, "shut up you old fool."

Mr. Charpentier's behavior gives the impression of an intense and all-absorbing state of withdrawal reflecting multiple aspects of the physical, emotional, and social dimensions. Physical indicators include staying in his room with physical retreat to one specific corner and repetitive hand movements. Vacant-looking eyes and preoccupation, including self-dialogue, seem indicative of an emotional withdrawal, whereas the social dimension is evident by avoidance behavior (e.g., avoidance of his roommate, other residents, and of social activities).

For Mr. Charpentier withdrawal initially was an active coping strategy, but it seems to have progressed to a more passive maladaptive behavior (evidenced by confusion and autistic behavior as emotional indicators) over the three years of residence. However, there definitely is an element of an active purposeful control strategy in the physical and social dimensions of withdrawal. Additionally, his degree of withdrawal seems greater than that of Mrs. Bianco, evidenced by the greater number of indicators and his extreme physical retreat with emergence of autistic behavior. Factors that seemed to influence the emergence of withdrawal for Mr. Charpentier include loss of control, length of time institutionalized, absent social support, inability to find a meaningful role, and physical variables of the environment itself.

Case 3—Mr. DuBois. Mr. DuBois is an 83-year-old widower of French Canadian descent who was referred to the researcher by a social worker as a new resident who may have difficulty adjusting. At the time of the researcher's initial encounter with Mr. DuBois, which was the second day after admission, there was no evidence of withdrawal.

Within the previous year, Mr. DuBois had experienced several losses, the most significant being the death of his wife. He was unable to maintain his own home and moved in with his son one month ago. Conflict developed with his daughter-in-law, "I felt like I was always in the way." Because he needed help with physical care, and could not maintain his own apartment, he agreed to relocate to a nearby nursing home. He was unhappy with the decision, yet realized there was little choice saying "I will try and make the best of it by just taking things as they come." He spoke positively of his son and grandson who would be visiting often.

During this initial encounter, Mr. DuBois looked relieved to see a friendly face. He spoke of his recent losses such as his wife, home, car, and his generally declining health due to osteoarthritis. Since his retirement at age 65, the majority of his leisure time was spent gardening and woodworking, which he still does on a limited basis. Throughout the conversation, he remained alert and attentive, maintaining eye contact and displaying facial expressions appropriate to the context of the topic (i.e., when he spoke of his wife, he looked sad).

The next encounter was five days after relocation. The researcher observed Mr. DuBois walking down the corridor. He seemed to have difficulty maneuvering within the environment, and when he reached the lounge, he sat in the first available chair. When the researcher approached him, he smiled saying that he was "happy to see a familiar face." The researcher shared with Mr. DuBois her observations concerning his hesitancy in moving about the nursing unit. He attributed his hesitancy to "being unfamiliar with the place," but felt that with time he would adjust because he was usually an adaptable, outgoing man. He remained attentive during the conversation relating that his son visited last evening and took him out for dinner.

The following week, Mr. DuBois was transferred to a smaller nursing home near his son's home. This facility had been his son's first choice. Two weeks later the researcher gained entry to this nursing home. Mr. DuBois was alone in the residents' lounge. Initially, he did not recognize the researcher, and he exhibited a decrease in eye contact and a lack of facial expression. He seemed indifferent to the researcher's presence relating that he was tired and was going to lie down on his bed. The researcher followed him to his room and found him lying down with his face averted toward the wall.

Interviews with the nursing staff led to some unsettling information. They described Mr. DuBois as a quiet, somewhat confused man who spent most of his time alone in his room. He did not interact socially with the other residents and occasionally got lost wandering within the nursing home. Nurses' notes included such comments as "keeps to himself, sleeps often especially during the day, potential for socialization not known at this time." One nurse related that he seemed a bit "withdrawn, and was taking some time to adjust." Attempts at getting Mr. DuBois involved in social activity were not very successful.

Subsequent observations on two occasions elicited similar data of daytime sleeping or sitting alone in the lounge. On a third encounter, when the researcher approached Mr. DuBois he got up from the chair and went toward his room saying that he was "tired and needed to lie down." He went outdoors, wandered around the yard saying he was "looking for his room." It seemed that Mr. DuBois was becoming more withdrawn. He was physically retreating to his room, sleeping more often during the day, and sometimes wandered about the nursing home. Emotionally, he had an apathetic affect and began to show signs of confusion. Social withdrawal seemed apparent by silence and avoidance of social interaction, particularly lack of interaction with the researcher.

After sharing these impressions with the staff, the researcher stayed with Mr. DuBois to talk with him. He related that he felt lonely, and wished that he was home with his wife. He still missed her terribly and had little desire to do anything. He could not get interested in the type of activities available in the nursing home. A meeting was held between the staff, activity director, and the researcher. Interventions were identified to increase Mr. DuBois's recognition of his room and minimize wandering. The activity director spent additional time assessing his interests, and plans were devised for Mr. DuBois to join a weekly social hour. Opportunities for gardening and the development of a woodworking shop were explored. The staff approached Mr. DuBois more often and spent considerable time increasing his interest.

Over time, these interventions led to a decrease in withdrawal behaviors. For example, he spent less time sleeping during the day, increased his interaction with other residents, became more talkative, made eye contact, exhibited facial expressions, and spoke positively about the upcoming Christmas holiday plans at his son's home. He also related that he was beginning to enjoy the social hour because he had an opportunity to speak French with some other men. On the final meeting day, the researcher attended a holiday party with Mr. DuBois who wore a bow tie and jokingly referred to the researcher as "his date."

For Mr. DuBois withdrawal was a passive, progressive maladaptive behavioral response to the stress of relocation. Without recognition and intervention, it was apparent that withdrawal would continue to progress. Factors that seemed to negatively affect Mr. DuBois's adjustment and contributed to his withdrawal included the recent loss of a significant other, compounded by other recent losses, the inability to find a meaningful role, and possible depression.

Final Analytical Phase

This fieldwork phase added empirical support to the existence and importance of withdrawal among nursing home residents. As in the literature, nurses in this study viewed withdrawal as mainly negative. Withdrawal was considered a nursing care problem that required intervention by increasing socialization. The field data did not fully support the idea that withdrawal was negative suggesting that nurses may need to be more attentive to the assumption that withdrawal is inherently problematic. Certainly, this researcher's initial impression that withdrawal is a negative phenomenon interfering with residents' adaptation to nursing home settings was challenged.

Among the residents studied here, withdrawal emerged most frequently as an active coping strategy, and also as a passive behavioral response. These two manifestations of withdrawal seem consistent with what was described in the literature, particularly with the types of withdrawal experiences found by Cochrane (1983). What was evident from this fieldwork, which was not apparent in the literature review, is the long-term continuous use of withdrawal as an active coping strategy. This was evidenced by Mrs. Bianco, somewhat by Mr. Charpentier, and in the case that was not presented. The variables of lifestyle, personality traits, and affective response to the nursing home environment itself seem most useful in explaining this continuous active withdrawal.

These residents had limited or no social support most of their lives. They perceived themselves as not socially outgoing, preferring to be alone to engage in individual activities including reminiscing. Generally, they denied feeling lonely or depressed. The avoidance of other residents and lack of participation in social activities as social indicators of withdrawal can be explained as follows. These residents lacked the social skills to participate in group activities. Consequently, the nursing home environment with its emphasis on socialization was incongruent with their personalities and reinforced the withdrawal. Additionally, the physical layout of the nursing home, with its close proximity to other residents, supported the physical withdrawal that has been illustrated by Tate (1980) as an attempt to secure personal space and privacy. Finally, emotional withdrawal as a form of mental disengagement, similar to the concept of conservation-withdrawal as described by Ironside (1980), protected them from the continuous emotional drain emanating from an environment inconsistent with their self-concept. Therefore, withdrawal emerged as an active coping strategy with positive effects and continued to be used to maintain control and cope with the stressors inherent in the nursing home environment.

In contrast to this manifestation of withdrawal, a passive and progressive withdrawal with negative effects was evident in Mr. DuBois that can be explained by the following analysis. Unlike the other residents studied, Mr. DuBois was a sociable man with an active support system prior to his wife's death and his relocation to his son's home. Since his recent losses of wife, home, and health, Mr. DuBois was faced with three consecutive relocations. The dramatic emergence and progression of withdrawal became evident during the stress of relocation to the second nursing home and was negatively influenced by the factors of minimal social support to buffer this stress, loss of control, and inability to find a meaningful role. Additionally, the self-reported feelings of loneliness and depression seem associated with the withdrawal. This negative response of withdrawal is comparable to a giving up syndrome or "resigned resistance" of the aged as described by Chenitz (1983).

Furthermore, although this study did not focus on nurse-patient inter-action, observations of the staff indicated that avoidance was a subtle, yet predominant interactional pattern that may have further reinforced Mr. DuBois's withdrawal. These observations emphasize the need to examine the potential of mutual withdrawal as encountered by Tudor (1952) be-tween nursing staff and nursing home residents. Further study may support the idea that withdrawal is most significant as a nurse-client related phe-nomenon and is best studied as an interactional concept.

Future investigations need to examine withdrawal as a progressive phe-nomenon and attempt to further delineate those factors that influence pro-gression. Additionally, closely related concepts and their potential inter-active effect could be examined. Depression and loneliness were concepts that indirectly emerged during unstructured interviewing in these cases and were identified in the literature as potential maladaptive behavioral re-sponses of the aged. The resident's subjective reports of the presence or absence of these feelings may begin to support an empirical generalization suggesting that loneliness and depression may contribute to a progressive withdrawal.

Findings confirmed earlier impressions of withdrawal as a retreat and supported the initial working definition to some extent. Yet, further expan-sion and refinement of the concept is needed to encompass the full meaning of withdrawal as both a *positive* strategy and a *negative* behavioral response. Furthermore, the initial definition focused on withdrawal as a behavioral response, implying passivity, rather than an active strategy. Therefore, the essential nature of withdrawal seems to be a multidimensional, bipolar con-cept that can be operationalized on a continuum ranging from adaptive coping behaviors to maladaptive behavioral responses. Following this the-oretical and empirical analysis, a refined working definition would be: With-drawal is a behavior characterized by physical, social, and emotional retreat from people, things, and/or situations. The retreat may be active and/or passive, which can be depicted on a continuum ranging from adaptation to maladaptation and can be measured through behavioral indicators. Addi-tionally, measures used in this fieldwork phase add empirical support to those behavioral indicators identified in Table 9−1. Although no additional indicators became evident, those of avoidance of people, including avoid-ance of social situations, and retreat to one's room were the most frequent in all cases. These findings support the need to further identify and measure these behavioral indicators.

Empirical observations in the fieldwork phase emphasize the need to examine the potential for withdrawal in other populations faced with con-tinuous stress. Those populations that merit inquiry include the chronically ill, long-term hospitalized, mentally ill and terminally ill client. Nurses could examine the stress associated with illness, yet also explore the impact of stress associated with relocation. Slavinsky and Krauss (1980) suggest that the problems associated with deinstitutionalization of the chronic mentally ill person can be explained by the concept of mutual withdrawal. The focus of study could be at the client level, nurse-client level, and client-community level in an effort to examine all potential interactive processes of withdrawal. Further inquiry might discover that withdrawal is a central phenomenon in nursing, common to most people as they attempt to deal with the anxiety associated with stressful situations. The crucial factor for nursing seems to be the discovery of when withdrawal is no longer adaptive and intervention is indicated.

In conclusion, the hybrid model of concept development was most useful in analyzing withdrawal for several reasons. First, it is an inductive process that facilitated the use of empirical observations of withdrawal in developing a definition and indicators for measuring this concept in nursing. Second, the flexibility of the model encouraged the researcher to move back and forth between the theoretical and fieldwork phase, continuously generating new insights, which in this case limited the premature conceptualization of withdrawal as an inherently negative phenomenon. Finally, and most importantly, the use of participant observation gave the researcher a richness of real life experience that was crucial for clarifying the concept of withdrawal, elucidating ideas on definition and measurement, and identifying variables influencing its emergence and progression.

REFERENCES

Andreasen, N. C., & Flaum, M. (1991). Schizophrenia: The characteristic symptoms. *Schizophrenia Bulletin, 17*(1), 27–49.

Achenbach, T. M., & Edelbrock, C. S. (1978). The classification of child psychopathology: A review and analysis of empirical efforts. *Psychological Bulletin, 85*(6), 1275–1301.

Ballard, K. D. (1983). The role of intervention frequency in identifying socially withdrawn and socially isolated children: A re-examination of data and concepts. *Educational Psychology, 3*(2), 115–126.

Beland, I. (1980). The burnout syndrome in nurses. In Werner-Beland, J. (Ed.), *Grief responses to long-term illness and disability; Manifestations and nursing interventions* (pp 189–213). Reston, Va: Reston.

Bleuler, E. (1912). *The theory of schizophrenic negativism* (Nervous and Mental Disease Monograph Series No. II). New York: The Journal of Nervous and Mental Disease.

Borup, J. H. (1983). Relocation mortality research: Assessment, reply, and the need to refocus on the issues. *The Gerontologists, 23*(3), 235–242.

Brehm, H. P. (1968). Sociology and aging: Orientation and research. *Gerontologist, 8,* 24–31.

Burbank, P. M. (1986). Psychosocial theories of aging: A critical review. *Advances in Nursing Science, 9*(1), 73–86.

Chenitz, C. E. (1983). Entry into a nursing home as status passage: A theory to guide nursing practice. *Geriatric Nursing, 4,* 92–97.

Cochrane, N. J. (1983). An explanatory study of social withdrawal experiences of adults. *Nursing Papers, 15*(2), 22–37.

Cumming, E., & Henry, W. E. (1961). *Growing old—The process of disengagement.* New York: Basic Books.

Daum, J. M. (1983). Emotional indicators in drawings of aggressive and withdrawn male delinquents. *Journal of Personality Assessment, 47*(3), 243–249.

Davis, M. Z. (1975). Social isolation as a process in chronic illness. In M. Z. Davis, M. Kramer, & A. L. Strauss (Eds.), *Nurses in practice: A perspective on work environments.* St. Louis: Mosby.

deLeon, J., Wilson, W. H., & Simpson, G. M. (1989). Measurement of negative symptoms in schizophrenia. *Psychiatric Developments, 3,* 211–234.

Edmunds, M. (1974). *Defences in animals: A survey of anti-predator defences.* New York: Longman.

Engel, G.L., & Reichsman, F. (1956). Spontaneous and experimentally induced depression in an infant with gastric fistula. *Journal of American Psychoanalytic Association, 4*(3), 428–452.

Fields, M. J. (1985). The analytic alliance: "Pre-empathic" interventions with withdrawn narcissistic patients. *Psychotherapy, 22*(3), 572–582.

Friedrick, R. M., & Lively, S. I. (1981). Psychological immobilization. In L. K. Hart, J. L. Reese, & M. O. Fearing (Eds.), *Concepts common to acute illness: Identification and management.* St. Louis: Mosby.

Frieswyk, S. (1977). The assessment of a relational disposition, "fantasy withdrawal" from Rorschach face sheet data. *Journal of Clinical Psychology, 33*(4), 1132–1140.

Glaser, B. G., & Strauss, A. L. (1965). *Awareness of dying.* Chicago: Aldine.

Greenwood, C. R., Walker, H. M., & Haps, H. (1977). Issues in social interaction: Withdrawal assessment. *Exceptional Children, 13*(8), 490–499.

Gurland, B. J., Dean, L. J., & Cross, P. S. (1983). The effects of depression on individual social functioning in the elderly. In L. D. Breslau & M. R. Haug (Eds.), *Depression and Aging: Causes, care and consequences.* New York: Springer Publishing.

Hamburg, D. A., Hamburg, B., & deGoza, S. (1953). Adaptive problems and mechanisms in severely burned patients. *Psychiatry, 16*(1), 1–21.

Hurteau, P. M. (1963). Disguised language: A clinical problem in nursing. In S. F. Burd & M. A. Marshall (Eds.), *Some clinical approaches to psychiatric nursing* (pp. 32–36). London: Macmillan.

Hutchinson, S. (1987). Self-care and job stress. *Image, 19*(4), 192–196.

Ironside, W. (1980). Conservation-withdrawal and action-engagement: On a theory of survivor behavior. *Psychosomatic Medicine, 42*(1:11), 163–175.

Jacobson, S. F. (1983). Burnout: A hazard in nursing. In S. F. Jacobsen & M. H. McGrath (Eds.), *Nurses under stress* (pp. 98–110). New York: John Wiley & Sons.

Jasmin, S., & Trygstad, L. N. (1979). *Behavioral concepts and the nursing process.* St. Louis: Mosby.

Kendler, K. S. (1985). Diagnostic approaches to schizotypal personality disorder: A historical perspective. *Schizophrenia Bulletin, 11*(4), 538–542.

Kim, M. J., McFarland, G. K., & McLane, A. M. (1987). *Pocket guide to nursing diagnoses* (2nd ed.). St. Louis: Mosby.

King, G. F. (1956). Withdrawal as a dimension of schizophrenia: An exploratory study. *Journal of Clinical Psychology, 12,* 373–375.

Kraepelin, E. (1904). *Lectures on clinical psychiatry.* Translated and edited by Thomas Johnstone. New York: Hafner.

Kramer, M. (1974). *Reality shock: Why nurses leave nursing.* St. Louis: Mosby.

Leyn, R. M. (1972). A mother's reaction to her son's fatal illness. *Maternal Child Nursing Journal, 13,* 231–241.

Lieberman, M. A., Prock, V. N., & Tobin, S. S. (1968). Psychological effects of institutionalization. *Journal of Gerontology, 23*(3), 343–353.

Lowenthal, M. F., & Boler, D. (1965). Voluntary vs. involuntary social withdrawal. *Journal of Gerontology, 20*(3), 363–371.

Maddox, G. L. (1965). Fact and artifact: Evidence bearing on disengagement theory from the Duke geriatrics project. *Human Development, 18,* 117–130.

McDonnell, T. E., & Beck, M. (1986). Temperament and psycho-social development. *Education, 106*(4), 413–418.

Moses, J. (1985). Stroking the child in withdrawn and disoriented elders. *Transactional Analysis Journal, 15*(2), 152–158.

O'Connor, R. D. (1969). Modification of social withdrawal through symbolic modeling. *Journal of Applied Behavior Analysis, 1*(2), 15–22.

Oden, G. (1963). Individual panic: Elements and patterns. In S. F. Burd & M. A. Marshall (Eds.), *Some clinical approaches to psychiatric nursing.* London: Macmillan.

Ollendick, T. H., Oswald, D. P., & Francis, G. (1989). Validity of teacher nominations in identifying aggressive, withdrawn, and popular children. *Journal of Clinical Child Psychology, 18*(3), 221–229.

Overall, J. E., & Gorham, D. R. (1962). The brief psychiatric rating scale. *Psychological Reports, 10,* 799–812.

Pallister, H. (1933). The negative or withdrawal attitude: A study in personality organization. *Archives of Psychology, 151,* 1–56.

Peplau, H. E. (1963). A working definition of anxiety. In S. F. Burd & M. A. Marshall (Eds.), *Some clinical approaches to psychiatric nursing.* London: Macmillan.

Ross, A. D., Lacey, H. M., & Parton, D. A. (1965). The development of a behavior checklist for boys. *Child Development, 36,* 1013–1027.

Sapirstein, M. R. (1948). *Emotional security.* New York: Crown.

Schatzman, L., & Strauss, A. L. (1973). *Field research: Strategies for a natural science.* Englewood Cliffs, NJ: Prentice-Hall.

Schmidt, C. S. (1981). Withdrawal behavior of schizophrenics: Application of Roy's adaptation model. *Journal of Psychiatric Nursing and Mental Health Services, 19*(11), 26–33.

Scully, R. (1980). Stress in the nurse. *American Journal of Nursing, 80*(5), 912–915.

Serbin, L. A., Lyons, J. A., Marchessault, K., & Schwartzman, A. E. (1987). Observational validation of a peer nomination technique for identifying aggressive, withdrawn, and aggressive/withdrawn children. *Journal of Consulting and Clinical Psychology, 55*(1), 109–110.

Slavinsky, A. T., & Krauss, J. B. (1980). Mutual withdrawal . . . or Gwen Tudor revisited. *Perspectives in Psychiatric Care, 18*(5), 194–203.

Spitz, R. A., & Wolf, K. M. (1946). "Anaclitic depression." In A. Freud, H. Hartman, and E. Kris (Eds.), *The Psychoanalytic Study of the Child,* vol 2. New York: International Universities Press.

Tate, J. (1980). The need for personal space in institutions for the elderly. *Journal of Gerontological Nursing, 6,* 439–447.

Thomas, A., & Chess, S. (1977). Temperament and development. New York: Brunner/Mazel.

Tissue, T. L. (1968). A Guttman scale of disengagement potential. *Journal of Gerontology, 23*(4), 513–516.

Tobin, S. S., & Lieberman, M. A. (1976). *Last home for the aged.* San Francisco: Jossey-Bass.

Tudor, G. E. (1952). A sociopsychiatric nursing approach to intervention in a problem of mutual withdrawal on a mental hospital ward. *Psychiatry, 15*(2), 193–217.

Wagner, E. E. (1978). Diagnostic applications of the hand test. In B. B. Wolman (Ed.), *Clinical diagnosis of mental disorders: A handbook.* New York: Plenum.

Weinstein, E. A., Kahn, R. L., & Slote, W. H. (1956). Withdrawal, inattention and pain asymbolia. *Archives of Neurology and Psychiatry, 74,* 235–248.

Ziegler, L. H. (1933). Hysterical fugues. *Journal of the American Medical Association, 101*(5), 571–576.

Chapter 10

Concept Clarification: Using the Norris Method in Clinical Research

NANCY R. LACKEY

*C*atherine Norris (1982) stated in the preface of her book that one of her goals "is to foster the development of increasingly meaningful descriptions of nursing phenomena. Out of these descriptions will come critical questions and hypotheses which nurses will need to explore. Out of these descriptions, nurses will ultimately build the base for a substantive body of knowledge for the discipline called nursing" (p. xv). Norris has developed a method of concept clarification that can be used by nurse researchers to clarify phenomena that are germane to the knowledge base of nursing. The components from such clarification, once operationalized, can be used as variables in studies. The results of these studies will ultimately form a solid foundation from which effective nursing interventions can be derived.

Nurses in a variety of settings and roles care for a very diverse clientele: from the homeless to the very affluent, from the newborn to the frail elderly, from the single individual to the extended family. Lindsey (1991) stated that only through research will the quality of care provided by nurses improve. According to Lindsey, there are three critical stages in the development of a scientific base and in the integration of research findings into practice. These stages are (1) generation of nursing knowledge, (2) utilization of research, and (3) evaluation of the effectiveness of the specific changes in practice (p. 93). Before nursing knowledge can be generated, concepts pertinent to each of these diverse settings and roles must be identified and clarified and the components of the concept derived from the clarification incorporated into research questions or hypotheses that ultimately will be tested in some type of research. Norris (1982) has derived a method of concept clarification that can be used to identify the components of a concept that ultimately can be used to generate nursing knowledge to form the basis of more effective care for the diverse clientele that nurses serve.

The overall purpose of this chapter is to review and discuss Norris's method of concept clarification and delineate how nurses can use this method in their research to generate nursing knowledge as a solid foundation for nursing care. Discussed in this chapter are Norris's philosophical underpinnings for her method of concept clarification, the method itself, and an example that will illustrate the utility of her method of concept clarification for research.

Philosophical Foundation of Norris's Method

Norris (1982) wrote that research in nursing has suffered due to the lack of a well-defined body of knowledge and, conversely, the body of knowledge suffered because nurses have not done appropriate descriptive work, particularly concept clarification. She believed that there were some very great differences between the descriptive research done in medicine and the descriptive research needed in nursing. According to Norris, the research that had been done in medicine utilized the psyche-soma dualistic model. As a result, separate or several theories were developed for each disease studied by medicine. Because these theories were not analyzed or synthesized, medicine tended to view human beings in terms of a mind-body dichotomy and failed to recognize humans as a unique whole. Norris (1982) believed that nursing functioned independently from medicine and was consistent with a "humanistic, holistic approach to individuals and communities" (p. 6).

Important components of the knowledge base of nursing are the concepts used in nursing theory and practice. According to Norris (1982) a concept is a "basic idea," an "abstraction of concrete events," and the "only means of connecting an empirical science to the 'real world' "; the term *concept* is the "word symbol, not the act itself" (p. 11). Nursing requires two types of concepts: "one that relates to abstract knowledge and knowing (such as the concept 'wellness'), and one that is process-oriented and answers questions about how to solve nursing problems" (such as cardiovascular fitness) (p. 13). The concepts of nursing knowledge and practice articulate the essence of nursing science; that science is dependent upon precise language to convey the phenomenon. The effective use of language requires the precision of adequate concept clarification. Norris stated that concepts are "generalizations about particulars, such as cause-effect, duration, dimension, attributes, and continua of phenomena or objects" (p. 11). The process of concept clarification allows us to make generalizations and to systematize the particulars. From these generalizations and systematizations, an operational definition of the concept can be derived. Operational definitions allow us to know when the concept under study is in operation, and thus, they can become the basis for research. Operational definitions, because of their preciseness, articulate the essence of nursing science.

In Norris's (1982) review of the history of concept clarification, it was apparent that very few researchers actually attempted an empirical approach to concept clarification. Norris believed that the only way to build nursing knowledge was by a systematic empirical process that should be applied without exception. Historically, the method of concept clarification used by nurses was focused on a review of the literature regarding a specific concept and then presented as a summary of that literature review. Norris concluded that the existing methods of concept clarification were inadequate and new methods were needed to produce operational definitions and conceptual models from which testable hypotheses could be devised. She proposed that (a) concepts explored generally in the past be studied to clarify their components and roles in specific situations, (b) current methodologies for concept clarification be refined and new methodologies be developed, and (c) nurses become familiar with various modes of synthesis. Attention to these three issues would expedite nursing research and, consequently, enhance the development of a body of knowledge for the profession.

Norris (1982) further believed that concept clarification without experimental research was ineffective because the method by itself could not fulfill the requirements of knowing. Similarly, she argued that "experimental research without concept clarification is meaningless" (p. 11). Consequently, Norris believed that concept clarification should culminate in an operational definition for use in further research. She advocated the development of a model of the concept that specified its components and the relationships among these components as a product of the inquiry. Such a model puts the concept into proper perspective with existing theories. Then, after the independent and dependent variables were identified, hypotheses could be derived that could be tested empirically. Based on these beliefs, Norris developed the following method of concept clarification.

Norris's Method of Concept Clarification

Nursing theory can be developed inductively, deductively, or through a combination of the two forms of inquiry. Norris believed that the inductive approach to theory development was based on empirical evidence and from clinical practice. She further believed that the inductive collection of data from practice identified behavioral phenomena that relate to human health, illness, and comfort, phenomena with which clients confronted nurses or that nurses anticipated. Using the inductive approach, a nursing phenomenon would be observed and analyzed. From the analysis, concepts could be constructed that explained the observed phenomenon. Models would be derived that would help to further explain the observed phenomenon.

The goal of Norris's method is to collect empirical data and analyze it in ways that increasingly build to higher levels of abstraction. As a result, theories of human behavior in health and illness could be constructed. Ultimately, nurses could understand, predict, and control phenomena. Inductive inference should begin with a specific case and move toward generalities until an inductively derived model would fit into one or more of the deductively constructed theories. In her discussion of concept clarification, Norris never discussed how her method could be used to develop nursing theory deductively or through a combination of the two forms of inquiry.

There are five steps in Norris's (1982) method of concept clarification:
1. After identifying the concept of interest, observe and describe the phenomena repeatedly and, if possible, describe the phenomena from the point of view of other disciplines.
2. Systematize the observations and descriptions.
3. Derive an operational definition of the concept under study.
4. Produce a model of the concept that includes all its component parts.
5. Formulate hypotheses.

The following is a description and discussion of each of the five steps of Norris's method of concept clarification.

OBSERVING AND DESCRIBING PHENOMENA

The purpose of the first step is to "describe, explain and give meaning to human behavior" (Norris, 1982, p. 16). This step begins with identification of the concept or phenomenon of interest. When the researcher has determined this focus of the inquiry, he or she then identifies and observes the phenomenon in a variety of clinical settings and describes, in detail, the sequence and context of events and the antecedents and consequences involved in the phenomenon. This description can either be written or tape-recorded for later transcription.

In this first step, the researcher also tries to identify examples of the phenomenon as it occurs in other disciplines. After speculating in what other disciplines the phenomenon might occur, the researcher consults representatives of those disciplines to determine if they have observed the phenomenon. For example, if the nurse researcher is studying the concept of abandonment, he or she may wish to consult with individuals in a department of social work. Social workers would be asked if they have seen the occurrence of this phenomenon and, if so, to give as complete a description as possible. This process enables the researcher to describe the phenomenon as completely as possible from a variety of perspectives. The researcher then records those varied descriptions of the phenomenon. After observing the phenomenon in as many situations and from as many relevant viewpoints as possible, the researcher conducts a thorough review of nursing and other literature to examine published reports of the occurrence of the phenomenon. The researcher thinks carefully about and reflects on all the possible meanings, relationships, sequences or orders, and causes and effects of the phenomenon in preparation for the second step, systematizing the observations.

SYSTEMATIZING THE OBSERVATIONS

After the researcher has pondered all the possible meanings, relationships, sequences, and causes and effects of the phenomenon, he or she begins to systematize the observations and descriptions. Norris (1982) defined systematization as "establishing categories, continua, hierarchies, and the like" (p. 16). She also stated that systematization activities include "observing, discovering, commonsense thinking, engaging in logical deduction and induction, searching for meaning, developing insights, testing out ways to organize, and speculating about types of relationships" (p. 19) that would help to further describe the concept under study. In this step the researcher is also looking for a sequence of events and for relationships to other events in the environment. Systematizing the observations involves classifying various aspects, components, or elements of the concept based on similarities and differences. The categories usually are based on properties of the concept, such as size, width, mass, bulk, color, capacity, location, temperature, time, frequency, duration, type, form, intensity, seriousness, and context in which the concept under study occurs. Categories are more valuable to researchers because they provide more information by indicating possible associational relationships. The following are some of the questions that might be asked during this step: In what type of situation did this phenomenon occur? What events triggered the phenomenon? Are there events that were triggered by the phenomenon itself? Are there certain patterns, categories, or a process that evolve as the phenomenon occurs? What happened as a result of the occurrence of this phenomenon? Upon completion of this step, the researcher should have an understanding of the scope and depth of the concept under study.

DEVELOPING AN OPERATIONAL DEFINITION

In the third step, an operational definition of the concept is formulated. Norris (1982) stated that an operational definition answers at least one question, "How will I know the concept when (in the broadest sense) I see it in operation?" (p. 16). Other views concerning operational definitions emphasize *measurement,* however. Chinn and Kramer (1991), for example, indicated specifically that an operational definition explicates ways to "measure" the behaviors observed in a phenomenon (p. 101). Similarly, Walker and Avant (1988) pointed out that an operational definition is the "means by which we can classify a phenomenon as an example of the concept . . . and . . . a means by which to measure the concept in question" (p. 138). Also emphasizing measurement, Waltz, Strickland, and Lenz (1991) indicated that "an operational definition provides meaning by defining a concept in terms of the observations and/or activities that measure it" (p. 34). The emphasis on measurement in operationalizing a concept is a significant outcome of concept clarification in that it provides a basis for future empirical research through the quantification of variables.

In her own study of nausea and vomiting, Norris (1982) identified three distinct stages of nausea and, consequently, created three operational definitions of the concept. Because she thought that there were no observable indicators of nausea in its early stage and that the experience was subjective, "early nausea" was operationally defined in regard to the verbal statements of individuals. Statements included the clients' expressed sensations:

- queasiness, uneasiness over the area of stomach, esophagus, and pharynx associated with the subject naming it "nausea"
- verbal statement by subject of heaviness, pressure, or sinking feeling over area of stomach or sternum associated with the subject naming it "nausea"
- verbal statement by subject of inclination to vomit (p. 99)

A second operational definition was proposed for the "late phase" of nausea (Norris, 1982). This definition combined signs and symptoms with the parasympathetic stimulation and indicated all of the manifestations of early nausea. In addition, the late phase of nausea also included:

- vasomotor changes, that is, diaphoresis, feeling of being hot or cold
- increased salivation (p. 101)

The last definition of nausea included:

- forced inspiration
- retching, that is, labored, rhythmic respiratory activity
- rhythmic contraction of abdominal muscles
- vomiting posture, that is, head and neck extended, mouth open (p. 101)

Finally, an operational definition of vomiting was provided:

- liquid and/or semisolid matter that represents the stomach contents is ejected through the mouth
- simultaneously with this ejection, the diaphragm and abdominal muscles contract in unison (p. 103)

Nevertheless, as Norris (1982) noted, the formulation of operational definitions may be difficult because of imprecision in the use of terms, lack of clarification of nursing phenomena, and the lack of discriminatory skills needed to identify relevant aspects of the concept of interest. Norris did not provide any insights as to how to rectify this issue.

CONSTRUCTING A MODEL

The fourth step is the construction of a model. The model gives meaning to the data by increasing the generalization about the concept and distinguishing the relationships among the various kinds of categories in some communicable way. Norris identified two functions of the model. First, it enables the researcher to reexamine the previously defined categories, continua, hierarchies, and so forth, that were developed in step 2 in order to move the concrete data to a higher level of abstraction or to increase the generalization of the data. The model also facilitates the recognition of relationships among the previously established categories of data (Norris, 1982). Although higher levels of abstraction require causal relationships, other types of relationships can be determined at this time, including independence-dependence, concomitance, concurrence, sequence, temporal rate of relationships, and outcomes.

Models generally are not precise but serve as a medium to convey the phenomenon to others. Models are not the "real thing" but are depictions of the concepts or phenomena that they represent. Models can be constructed in many forms, including the use of mathematical symbols or physical materials, such as a model of human anatomy. In some instances, a combination of forms may be used to construct the model (Chinn & Kramer, 1991). Often, the more abstract the phenomenon, the more difficult it is to develop a model.

DEVELOPING HYPOTHESES

The last step of concept clarification according to Norris (1982) is hypothesis formation. A hypothesis is a statement that predicts a relationship between two or more variables and is derived directly from the model. Hypotheses are formed by the questions that the model creates, the inconsistencies observed, and the inadequacies or "holes" in the schematic representation. The researcher does an in-depth analysis of the relationships within the model to determine which ones, if any, are already supported by empirical research and which of the relationships need further study. Hypotheses based on these relationships and observations can then be tested using experimental research methods. Norris (1982) stressed that the "role of research is paramount in confirming or refuting whether categories assigned and whether causal, coexistence, or sequential relationships exist" (p. 35).

An Example of Concept Clarification Using Norris's Method

While a graduate student in 1989, Marilyn Stockdale wanted to learn more about Norris's method of concept clarification and to be a part of the research program. Since Norris's research program revolved around identifying the needs of various groups of clinical patients, Stockdale used this method to clarify the concept *human needs.* Nurses in all clinical areas deal with human needs, and this concept is fundamental to the nature and scope of nursing. Yet this concept had not been clarified for use in the profession. What is a human need? How does one distinguish between the individual concepts of need, problem, goal, want, wish, or desire? Are there levels of human needs and, if so, which levels should nurses be dealing with? The following describes the process used by Stockdale (1989) and her findings.

STEP 1: OBSERVING AND DESCRIBING THE PHENOMENON

The first step is to observe and describe the phenomenon repeatedly and if possible describe it as it occurs in other disciplines (Norris, 1982). Stockdale had observed patients in her clinical practice with various needs that she classified as "human needs," and she described in detail several of these situations. She also knew that this phenomenon existed in other disciplines. Instead of approaching individuals in these varied disciplines and asking them to describe the phenomenon, she conducted an integrative review of the literature. A cursory review of the literature indicated that the concept occurred and had been the focus of literature in nursing and many other disciplines over the years but that there had not been any agreement on a specific taxonomy or classification or on an operational definition of the concept.

Stockdale (1989) made the following assumptions about the concept of human needs:

- All human beings have needs.
- Humans experience needs which have subjective meaning and importance.
- Needs change and have varying degrees of urgency and strength.
- Needs are not always recognized or acknowledged by the individual.
- Significant deprivation of needs will result in physiological and/or psychosocial harm.
- Nursing intervention has the potential to improve the well being of the human condition.
- Need theory is applicable to all aspects of nursing practice (p. 7).

Stockdale (1989) also found writings from several disciplines that addressed the concept of human needs. As Lederer (1980) noted, the fields of psychology, sociology, philosophy, biology, anthropology, economics, as well as other disciplines, all have contributed to the study of human needs. Similarly, Stockdale found the range of theoretical approaches to the concept of human needs to be very diverse. She found that *need* and *problem* were two different concepts but that they were frequently used interchangeably in the literature. Stockdale cited Block (1974) as stating that because these concepts are used in the nursing process and because many states use these two terms in their nurse practice acts, it was important for nurses to agree on their meanings and use the concepts consistently.

In her review of literature Stockdale reported that there were four established theories of needs. The earliest of these was proposed by Murray

(1938), who postulated that human behavior is attributed to the force of need from within as:

> *a construct (a convenient fiction or hypothetical concept) which stands for a force (the physio-chemical nature of which is known) in the brain region, a force which organizes perception, apperception, intellection, connotation, and action in such a way as to transform in a certain direction an existing unsatisfying situation. (pp. 123–124)*

Murray thought the concept of need was closely related to the concept of drive, and subsequently identified two types of needs. Primary or viscerogenic needs were described as basic in nature and included needs for air, water, food, sex, lactation, urination, defecation, harm-avoidance, heat-avoidance, cold-avoidance, and sentience. Secondary needs were described as dependent on primary needs and included common reaction systems and wishes, such as nurturance.

Maslow's (1954) theory of the hierarchy of needs is perhaps one of the best known of all the need theories. Maslow's theory of motivation included a five-level hierarchical structure of basic needs that incuded physiological needs as the most fundamental, followed by safety, belongingness and love, esteem, and self-actualization. The gratification of each stage of needs submerged them and allowed the next higher set of needs to emerge. Unsatisfied physiological needs dominate an individual, whereas higher levels of needs are less imperative for survival and produce more desirable subjective results within the human being.

A theory of existence, relatedness, and growth needs was developed by Alderfer (1972). Alderfer thought there was no reason to distinguish between desire, satisfaction, and need and defined needs as "a concept subsuming both desires and satisfactions (frustrations)" (p. 8). In his theory, existence needs were a person's requirement for the exchange of material and energy to reach and maintain equilibrium with regard to material substances. Relatedness needs acknowledged that a person must engage in an interaction with the environment. Growth needs originated from the tendency of open systems to increase in internal order and differentiation over time as a result of interacting with the environment.

The last theory of needs reviewed by Stockdale was a nursing human need theory developed by Yura and Walsh (1988). These authors applied the concept of human needs to the nursing process and subsequently constructed a theory for use with what they proposed to be basic concepts in nursing: person, family, and community. In their theory, 35 human needs were identified and categorized into survival, closeness, or freedom needs. Human need was defined as a fulfillment of a state in which a person experiences satisfaction of the need with the approximate or target satisfier in an amount sufficient to create a wellness state for the person.

Several other works that specifically addressed the concept of need were discovered by Stockdale as well. Etionzini (1984), for example, suggested there is a universal set of human needs that have attributes of their own and that are not determined by social structure, cultural patterns, or socialization processes. He differentiated between those needs that were shared with the animal kingdom and those that he thought were uniquely human such as affection and recognition. Montagu (1951), however, viewed humans as animals that must breathe, eat, drink, excrete, sleep, maintain adequate health, and procreate. Basic needs were defined by Montagu as "any urge or need which must be satisfied if the organism or the group is to survive" (p. 51). However, Montagu also pointed out that humans have other needs, such as emotions or biological urges, that are not necessary for physical survival but that must be satisfied if the person is to develop and maintain adequate mental health. According to Stockdale (1989), the needs identified by Montagu dealt with acquired needs that grow out of the person's relation to derived or socially emergent needs. Although these needs are not necessary for survival, they are necessary for maintaining mental health.

Galtung (1980) similarly defined needs as "a necessary condition, as something that has to be satisfied at least to some extent in order for the need-subject to function as a human being" (p. 3). Nevertheless, this author categorized needs into four broad categories: security, welfare, identity, and freedom.

In nursing, the works of Peplau and Roy were found to have made a substantial contribution to the understanding of human needs (Stockdale, 1989). Peplau (1952), a nurse theorist, developed a framework for psychodynamic nursing based on the psychology of personality. Peplau saw nurses as helpers who assisted clientele to meet their needs by providing certain specific conditions. For example, Peplau identified primary needs such as food, drink, rest, and sleep and also noted that secondary needs existed, including human needs for prestige, power, or participation with others. She believed that individuals alone know what their needs are, yet they may not be able to recognize or articulate them.

Roy (1976) defined need as a "requirement within the individual which stimulates a response to maintain integrity" (p. 15). Stockdale listed the needs that Roy identified as the basis for physiological integrity. These were exercise and rest, nutrition, elimination, fluid and electrolytes, oxygen, circulation and regulation, temperature, the senses, and the endocrine system. According to Stockdale (1989), Roy stated that as internal and external environments change, so does the degree of satiety.

Norris (1982) stated that in this first step the phenomenon under study should not be observed and described only from nursing's point of view but that it should be studied from the viewpoints of various disciplines. Stockdale, realizing that the concept of human needs was a pertinent concept for many disciplines, decided to do an extensive review of the literature to determine how the concept was described in other disciplines. This adaptation of Norris's method is very useful, appropriate, and economical of time for highly abstract concepts that are widely used in other disciplines, especially if there have been attempts by individuals in other disciplines to clarify the particular concept.

STEP 2: SYSTEMATIZATION AND DESCRIPTION

The second step in Norris's method, systematizing the observations and descriptions, is a cognitive process, thus difficult to demonstrate on paper. It involves rereading both the descriptions of the phenomenon given by workers in various clinical settings and the selected literature several times. As the researcher becomes immersed in the descriptions and literature, he or she begins to see patterns, categories, or hierarchies emerge. As the researcher looks for the categories, a definition tends to form.

As Stockdale carried out this step, she was able to identify two categories of needs: universal, or basic human needs, and needs that are unique to the individual. It was during this step of clarification that Stockdale identified a pattern: The fulfillment of needs is a process that is in continuous operation within the individual. As she continued with Norris's method of concept clarification, she developed further insights regarding the concept and repeatedly returned to this step, reexamining her categories, and refining the derived patterns. During this process, Stockdale realized that the steps were not mutually exclusive but often needed to be carried on concurrently.

STEP 3: OPERATIONAL DEFINITION

According to Norris (1982), "the goal of concept clarification was to derive an operational definition" (p. 16). Because of the imprecision in the use of terms, lack of clarification of the phenomenon, and lack of discriminatory skills, it may be difficult for the researcher to construct an operational definition. Stockdale (1989) found this to be true as she reviewed the vast amount of literature about the concept of human needs. She did not find an operational definition of the concept in the literature review. Stockdale (1989) proposed the following definition of human needs applicable to nurses for clinical practice:

> *Human need is defined as a process of regulating survival, closeness, and freedom requirements. These may be partially fulfilled by the individual or a provider to prevent disequilibrium which is manifested in illness or maladjustment states. The extent that significant needs are restored is dependent on available resources and functional ability of the individual or society to receive the appropriate intervention. Satisfaction of human needs is based on subjective evaluation by the individual. (p. 43)*

Forming an operational definition is a cognitive process. This definition was formed based on the results of step 2, systematization and description. The categories and patterns derived were reviewed, and statements were formed that began to link these together. The definition was rewritten several times until the researcher thought it reflected the categories, patterns, and hierarchies derived from the observations made and the review of the literature.

STEP 4: MODEL

The fourth step in Norris's method is the production of a model. As previously stated, models help give meaning to the data by increasing the generalization about the concept and distinguishing the relationships among the categories, patterns, and hierarchies that have been derived. A well-constructed model should enhance communication of the results of a concept clarification. Stockdale (1989) proposed a model that depicted the impact that nursing has on meeting the needs of individuals within society. In Stockdale's model of human needs, nursing is seen as a force that diagnoses and treats human needs. In Figure 10–1, nursing is encased within a rectangle and the bold arrow depicts the force. The human being is seen as complex and holistic and is represented by the large circle at the center of this figure. Central to the internal structure of the human being are human needs. The pyramidal shape, outlined by arrows, illustrates the changing priority and urgency of the needs. These needs are interrelated with changing survival, closeness, and freedom needs. Stockdale further explained that external to a human are forces within society that also change and affect human needs. These forces are represented by a series of interrupted arrows surrounding the circle designated as man. The long arrows on the sides, showing a connection between the box labeled nursing and society represent the direct impact nursing has on society through its relationships with people. The outermost oval shape represents the world community; the bidirectional arrow between nursing and this world community reflects the global orientation of nursing in its interaction with people, an interaction that ultimately reaches the whole community of human beings.

STEP 5: HYPOTHESIS FORMATION

Norris (1982) stated that "testing the hypothesis moves the work into the experimental mode, where conclusions are stated with more certainty—that is, one learns whether the hypothesis was or was not supported by the results" (p. 18). Hypotheses are derived from the operational definition and the model. Following are some of the hypotheses that could be developed based on Stockdale's (1989) operational definition and model: the diagnosis of cancer does not change the number of human needs that an individual has; the extent to which some of the significant needs of patients with cancer can be met is dependent on their knowledge of available resources; the greater the decrease in functional ability of the patient with cancer, the

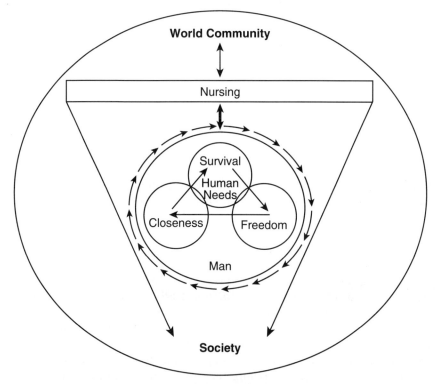

Figure 10–1 Stockdale's Proposed Model of Human Needs.
Reprinted with permission from Stockdale, M. (1989). *Human needs: Toward theory, conceptual clarification, and application to nursing.* Unpublished master's project, University of Kansas, Kansas City, Mo., p. 45.

greater the survival needs; closeness needs of patients with cancer who attend a cancer support group are not as great as those of patients who do not attend a cancer support group; and patients with cancer who are scheduled to see a clinical nurse specialist each time they come for their clinic appointments have more of their needs met than do those patients with cancer who do not see a clinical nurse specialist every time they come for their clinic appointments.

After the hypotheses are derived from the operational definition or the model, they are subjected to empirical testing. Such testing will either accept or reject the hypotheses. The operational definition and model derived from the process of concept clarification can then be revised to reflect the outcomes of such testing and, then, more hypotheses can be developed for empirical testing. This process continues until the researcher is satisfied that the operational definition and model really do describe the phenomenon under study.

Summary

Norris (1982) has stated,

> *In that nursing seeks to describe, clarify, predict, and control certain aspects of the world in which nurses work, it can be classified as an empirical, rather than a nonempirical, science. All advances in science require clarifying and relating the basic ideas involved. Specifically, advances in nursing science require clarifying the basic ideas in nursing and relating them to nursing's unique purposes, perspective, and universe of discourse (p. 12).*

In this chapter, Norris's five steps of concept clarification—(1) observing and describing phenomena, (2) systematizing and description, (3) developing an operational definition, (4) constructing a model, and (5) developing hypotheses—have been defined and described. An example using this method has been presented.

There are some strengths and weaknesses inherent in Norris's method. One of the strengths of her method is that it is described in five succinct steps. However, while using her method to clarify a very abstract concept, I frequently wanted more detail as to how one carried out some of the steps. For example, exactly how is an operational definition constructed from the systematization of the observations and descriptions identified in step 2? Her description of the five steps gives the reader the impression that each step is completed before the next is begun. In actuality, as the investigator goes through the process, he or she finds that the tentative conclusions developed in a step need to be substantiated by the previous step. For example, while trying to derive categories of needs in step 2, Stockdale (1989) had to return to step 1 and reexamine certain relationships and even review her original observations and literature. She repeated this process several times before she was able to complete step 2. This author found the method difficult to use while trying to clarify more abstract phenomena and believes that it can be used more effectively with those phenomena that are more observable (Chinn & Kramer, 1991), such as hemoglobin or nausea and vomiting.

I believe that Norris's (1982) method of concept clarification is relevant and can be used by nurse researchers to define and describe those phenomena that are an important part of nursing's diverse practice. When this occurs, gaps in nursing's scientific body of knowledge will be eliminated.

REFERENCES

Alderfer, C. P. (1972). *Existence, relatedness, and growth: Human needs in organizational settings.* New York: Free Press.

Block, D. (1974). Some crucial terms in nursing: What do they really mean? *Nursing Outlook, 22,* 689–694.

Chinn, P. L., & Kramer, M. K. (1991). *Theory and nursing: A systematic approach.* St. Louis: Mosby—Year Book.

Etionzini, A. (1984). Basic human needs, alienation, and inauthenticity. *American Sociological Review, 49,* 870–884.

Galtung, J. (1980). The basic needs approach. In K. Lederer (Ed.), *Human needs* (pp. 55–125). Cambridge, Mass: Oelgeschlager, Gunn, & Hain.

Lederer, K. (Ed.). (1980). *Human needs.* Cambridge, Mass: Oelgeschlager, Gunn, & Hain.

Lindsey, A. M. (1991). Integrating research and practice. In M. A. Mateo & K. T. Kirchhoff (Eds.), *Conducting and using nursing research in the clinical setting* (pp. 93–107). Baltimore: Williams & Wilkins.

Maslow, A. H. (1954). *Motivation and personality.* New York: Harper & Brothers.

Montagu, A. (1951). *On being human.* New York: Henry Schuman.

Murray, H. A. (1938). *Explorations in personality.* New York: Oxford University Press.

Norris, C. M. (1982). *Concept clarification in nursing.* Rockville, Md: Aspen.

Peplau, H. (1952). *Interpersonal relations in nursing: A conceptual framework of reference for psychodynamic nursing.* New York: Putnam.

Roy, S. C. (1976). *Introduction to nursing: An adaptation model.* Engelwood Cliffs, NJ: Prentice-Hall.

Stockdale, M. (1989). *Human needs: Toward theory, conceptual clarification, and application to nursing.* Unpublished masters project, University of Kansas, Kansas City, Mo.

Walker, L. O., & Avant, K. C. (1988). *Strategies for theory construction in nursing.* Norwich, Conn: Appleton & Lange.

Waltz, C. F., Strickland, O. L., & Lenz, E. R. (1991). *Measurement in nursing research.* Philadelphia: Davis.

Yura, H., & Walsh, M. B. (1988). *The nursing process: Assessing, planning, implementing, evaluating.* Norwalk, Conn: Appleton & Lange.

Chapter 11

Simultaneous Concept Analysis: A Strategy for Developing Multiple Interrelated Concepts

JOAN E. HAASE, NANCY KLINE LEIDY, DORIS D. COWARD, TERESA BRITT, AND PATRICIA E. PENN

S ystematic concept clarification and differentiation are critical to the advancement of knowledge and the development of scientific disciplines. The clear delineation of concepts is prerequisite to the evolution of theory, the development of measurement techniques, and the generation and testing of hypotheses. It is also necessary for clear, precise communication among members of the discipline.

Unfortunately, many concepts of concern to nurses are difficult to define and operationalize. Compounding these problems are issues of multidimensionality within single concepts and interrelatedness among multiple concepts. As a result, there are troublesome overlaps in definition and meaning, difficulties distinguishing between concepts, and, frequently, the inconsistent and inappropriate use of terminology. Coherent language, a uniform system of symbols that enables people to communicate intelligibly with one another, is critical to the development of any discipline. Thus, problems in terminology and concept clarification are obstacles to the development of the profession and science of nursing. Methods must be developed for the articulation of nursing concepts, removing as much ambiguity as possible and enabling clear communication among theorists, scientists, practitioners, and clients.

The purpose of this chapter is to describe a strategy of simultaneous concept analysis (SCA) designed to extend the clarification process origi-

This chapter is an extension of a paper titled "Concept Clarification using Consensus Group Process and Validity Matrices" presented February, 1991, at the Qualitative Health Research Conference, Edmonton, Alberta, Canada.

nally proposed by Wilson (1969) and introduced to nursing by Walker and Avant (1988). The strategy employs consensus group process and validity matrices to develop multiple interrelated concepts simultaneously. The purpose of SCA is to achieve clearer conceptual definitions, greater understanding of the meaning of individual concepts and the processes that may underlie their antecedents and outcomes, and insight into the interrelationships that exist among phenomena.

Thoughts on Independent Concept Analysis

Strategies have been developed for the systematic analysis of independent concepts. Wilson (1969) provided much of the groundwork for Walker and Avant's (1988) discussion of concept analysis for the construction of nursing theory. Their procedure includes such useful steps as determining the defining attributes of a selected concept, identifying antecedents and consequences, and defining empirical referents, among others. The limiting factor in this process, however, is its failure to suggest a method for considering, simultaneously, other similar or related concepts.

For example, in an analysis of the concept of spirituality, such as that proposed by Burkhardt (1989), questions are raised as to the extent to which defining attributes and outcomes of spirituality are adequately defined, in and of themselves. Burkhardt's description of harmonious interconnectedness as a defining characteristic is compelling, and intuitively meaningful for nursing. It is a critical component of her concept of spirituality, assuming roles as both a descriptive characteristic and a consequence. Nevertheless, harmonious interconnectedness remains undeveloped in a single concept analysis. By analyzing this concept simultaneously with spirituality, a greater understanding of the characteristics of the concept as well as the interrelationships of the processes of spirituality and harmonious interconnectedness can be attained.

The linkages between relevant concepts are as important to nursing as the static definitions of the concepts themselves. Is it not the dynamic, everchanging nature of human beings that is the focus of nursing intervention? Individual concept analysis is an excellent initiation into the identification and clarification of concepts relevant to nursing. Additional strategies, however, are needed to capture the breadth of individual concepts, to clarify the interrelationships with other concepts, and to begin to tap the dynamic nature of the processes that underlie nursing-relevant phenomena.

Simultaneous Concept Analysis

Through the strategy of SCA, concepts relevant to nursing can be more fully developed. In SCA, individual analyses of two or more concepts are accompanied by a critical examination of interrelated antecedents, defining characteristics, and outcomes. This examination leads to the development of definitions that are, by design, unique for each concept. At the same time, interrelationships and distinguishing elements across the concepts' antecedents, critical attributes, and outcomes are highlighted. The goal of this strategy is to gain insight into the potential sources of theoretical, empirical, and practical confusion among concepts, as well as offer greater understanding of the processes that might underlie each phenomenon.

In the remainder of this chapter, the procedures, peculiarities, and precautions of SCA are described. Examples from the author's experiences in developing and using this strategy will be presented. Specifically, the simultaneous analysis of the following four concepts will be discussed: spiritual perspective, hope, acceptance, and self-transcendence. A more detailed description of these concepts and the results of the SCA have been reported elsewhere (Haase, Britt, Coward, Leidy, & Penn, 1992).

THE SCA STRATEGY

Development of the SCA strategy was a group project that evolved over time. The following steps, perhaps more aptly called "sequence of events," became clear in retrospect. Because the evolution of ideas and group processes cannot be condensed to simple steps or a cookbook recipe, these steps are presented as guidelines to be used iteratively and flexibly. Readers may find them most useful when adjusted to the level, goals, and personality of the group involved. In general the steps used in SCA are as follows:

1. Development of the consensus group
2. Selection of concepts to be analyzed
3. Refinement of the concept clarification approach
4. Clarification of individual concepts
5. Development of validity matrices
6. Revision of individual concept clarifications
7. Reexamination of validity matrices
8. Development of a process model
9. Submission of the SCA results to peers for critique

Each of these steps will be discussed below. For clarification, we have included descriptions of some of our experiences with the development and use of the SCA strategy.

Development of the Consensus Group. The initial step in SCA is the formation of a consensus group, a set of individuals who are not only interested in several interrelated concepts, but are also capable of working independently and as a group, and are able to continue working together for a reasonable period of time, usually at least a year, to yield the desired outcome. We believe these are critical characteristics of the group and necessary for successful SCA.

Perhaps the greatest advantage of using a consensus group process in SCA is the diversity of perspectives contributing to the final product. Each individual brings a certain expertise to the group—a familiarity with use of the concept, knowledge of relevant literature, and representations of the concept in clinical practice. As will be discussed below, each individual uses this expertise to clarify a single concept, bringing ideas back to the group for discussion. Then, group members contribute their own perspectives and expertise to yield a product that reflects a consensus.

Individual expertise, together with a willingness to compromise and contribute, forms the foundation of the group. It is also helpful, although perhaps not necessary, to include a member who is interested in all concepts and the nature of their interrelationships, but is not necessarily committed to or invested in any single concept. This individual can serve as a group moderator, an unbiased participant who attempts to see both the forest and the trees and facilitates the group's journey along the most productive path.

A healthy alliance of qualitative and quantitative orientations within the group seems to broaden its perspective and promote creativity. Members with expertise in qualitative research guide the group toward meaning by encouraging depth, offering case studies, and considering philosophical implications. Complementing this orientation, the empiricists encourage the group to consider concrete issues, questioning the implications of SCA findings for operationalizing and testing concepts. A pleasant incidental is the understanding group members obtain from the two perspectives, and the tendency to integrate this understanding into individual theory development and research practices.

In our experience with SCA, several factors motivated the formation of a group to study the four concepts of spirituality, hope, acceptance, and self-transcendence. First, overlapping research interests led to frequent informal discussion on the definitions and meanings of various concepts we felt were important to nursing, yet elusive to empirical understanding. Similarly, we were all experiencing difficulty identifying and developing adequate measures for these complex, multidimensional concepts. Finally, we each felt that methods to operationalize these concepts for nursing must be devised. In order to develop these methods, however, clear and accurate theoretical descriptions of the concepts had to be developed.

We began meeting on a biweekly basis to help one another develop individual concept analyses and to compare and contrast the results. The group met regularly for over one year, with the membership remaining unchanged throughout this period. The products of those meetings were refined definitions for each concept, identification of the specific elements of each concept and their sequence of occurrence, clarification of interrelationships, and development of the SCA strategy.

Selection of Concepts to Be Analyzed. The second step in simultaneous concept analysis is to select the concepts to be analyzed. In reality, steps one and two are interrelated. Group formation arises out of common interests, and those interests drive concept selection. What must be realized, however, is the extent to which interests can vary, and be spirited on by group discussion and mutual intrigue.

To this point, we have presented the examples of spiritual perspective, hope, acceptance, and self-transcendence as though they were easily and decisively chosen. In reality, they represent four of many concepts we discussed, including courage, self-actualization, resilience, spirituality, and other, similar concepts that lie at the heart of our common research interests: health and adaptation in chronic illness. Through discussion and group consensus, the four concepts were chosen to best represent the most important, interrelated, and elusive of our interest areas. With time, it was discovered that some of the other concepts of interest seemed to be subsumed in these four. (Whether this "discovery" reflected a bias inadvertently introduced into the SCA by the group members, and therefore represents a limitation of the method, is an interesting discussion question.)

Refinement of the Concept Clarification Approach. After selecting the concepts to be analyzed, the next step in SCA is to determine the specific concept clarification techniques to be used. Factors to be considered include the extent to which (1) group members are familiar with specific techniques, (2) one technique is expressly preferred over another, (3) certain techniques are believed to be most effective in a group setting, or most effectively modified to meet group needs, and (4) efficiency is a priority since group process can be more protracted than independent work and, in some cases, certain deadlines (manuscripts, grants, and graduation, for example) must be met.

The group must reach a consensus and a sound understanding of the technique and terminology to be used in the individual concept clarification process (step 4). It may, in fact, take several sessions to reach this understanding. Nevertheless, it is imperative that each group member understand and use the same approach in order to permit later cross-concept comparisons.

In our analyses, we primarily used Wilson's (1969) concept clarification method. Several group meetings were spent discussing the basics of the method so that each member had a good understanding of the meaning of *antecedent, critical attribute,* and *outcome.* As we became immersed in the process, we found the need to devote time during later sessions to reclarification and redefinition of the approach selected. We also made the decision that it would be more efficient and effective to conduct case identification (i.e., model, related cases, and contrary cases as described by

Wilson) informally during group discussion, rather than by the individual responsible for a given concept analysis. This permitted all group members to contibute examples of cases derived from clinical, research, and personal experiences during group discussion. It also proved to be one of the more insightful and interesting aspects of the discussions.

Clarification of Individual Concepts. The fourth step in simultaneous concept clarification is the clarification of individual concepts. Each concept is initially analyzed by the respective expert. Working independently, the expert drafts preliminary definitions, critical attributes, antecedents, and outcomes based on a thorough review of existing theoretical and empirical literature, clinical experience, empirical data, and, when appropriate and useful, lay literature. Individuals may also employ expert consultants to assist in concept clarification.

The written "drafts" are discussed and critiqued in a group setting. Group members attempt to apply the concept in the context of their own knowledge base and clinical experiences. Any missing or unnecessary elements and any discrepancies or disagreements about what elements should be included in the concept are discussed and debated. Based on group feedback, each draft is rewritten by the individual expert and discussed in subsequent group sessions until all group members feel the definitions, antecedents, critical attributes, and outcomes contain the critical and the essential elements. That is, this process continues until the group reaches consensus on each concept analysis.

In our experience, it took several months to accomplish the individual analyses of the four concepts. Each meeting was devoted to one concept, considered as "le concept du jour." Adequate time (one to two hours) was necessary to allow the discussion to build momentum and decrease the time spent rehashing or reviewing previously addressed issues. We found that fewer meetings of longer duration, though more difficult to schedule, were the most effective and efficient strategy. Following the meeting, the draft was reworked independently by the respective expert, while the group rotated to another concept for the subsequent discussion.

In retrospect, it became apparent that we were becoming involved in a simultaneous concept analysis. Throughout each discussion, concepts were considered in light of the others. For example, while discussing self-transcendence as an outcome of hope, consideration was given to the critical attributes of self-transcendence discussed in an earlier meeting. Similarly, when energy was identified as a critical attribute of acceptance, consideration was given to this attribute in hope and spiritual perspective. This is a strength of SCA and the rationale behind using group process during the individual concept clarification step of this strategy.

During the individual clarification stage, we made several observations about group process that may be helpful to others using SCA or other similar approaches. First, challenges to assertions were done in respectful and valuing ways. Second, the individual doing the initial work on the concept was considered the expert. The group would push that person hard for clarification or justification of their work. We expected challenges to be met through specific theoretical writings, research, case examples, and other acceptable references.

Third, debate was not concluded until all group members felt the essence of the idea was complete and accurate based on the available theoretical, empirical, and experiential knowledge base. The massive amounts of information we were juggling forced us to deal with only essential elements. There were times, however, when the expert was heavily invested in the concept during this phase, and the group had to work diligently to eliminate all but the essential elements. We often felt that to achieve theoretical parsimony, some of the interesting and rich subtleties of a concept were put aside. In the interest of breadth, understanding, and a glimpse at the processes underlying multiple concepts simultaneously, individuals learned to let go of certain aspects of "their" concept, for the time being, and to continue the analysis process.

Fourth, although several individuals were consulted about specific concepts during this phase of the process, consultants were not included in group discussion. Again in retrospect, limiting meetings to the work group contributed to its cohesiveness and enhanced group process. The use of consultants, however, strengthened the group's knowledge base and enhanced its image as scholarly, open, and task-oriented.

Finally, all group members contributed to the background information necessary for individual concept analysis. Individuals shared their knowledge of the literature, philosophical bases, and clinical or personal experiences. Each source was considered legitimate and highly valued by the group. All sources of knowledge were critically evaluated before being accepted as valid.

Results of Individual Concept Clarification. The results for this step in the SCA strategy are, simply stated, definitions, critical attributes, antecedents and outcomes with supporting references for each concept. Figure 11–1 displays the antecedents, critical attributes, and outcomes we identified for one of the concepts analyzed in our group, spiritual perspective. At this point, disregard the boxes, arrows, and bold print. The realization of these elements came much later in the SCA process.

For illustrative purposes, let us examine this concept in more detail. The few words in Figure 11–1 do not convey the depth of discussion that preceded this version of the concept analysis. For example, notice that spirituality is considered an antecedent. Although *spirituality* is the term most frequently found in the literature, and the term we were using at the

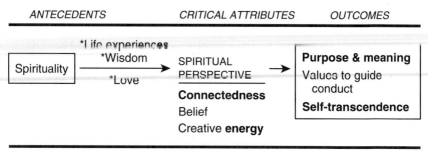

ANTECEDENTS   CRITICAL ATTRIBUTES   OUTCOMES

*Life experiences
*Wisdom

Spirituality ───────► SPIRITUAL   **Purpose & meaning**
*Love   PERSPECTIVE   Values to guide
                                            conduct
                         Connectedness **Self-transcendence**
                         Belief
                         Creative **energy**

*   Enablers
──►   Indicates the direction of the process
Bold   Indicates that the element occurs more than once

Figure 11–1 Process model for spiritual perspective.

beginning of the SCA process, group discussion yielded a consensus that spirituality was a basic or inherent quality of all humans. We concluded that the phenomenon that varies between individuals is spiritual perspective, a highly individualized awareness of one's spirituality and its qualities. Notice, too, that love, knowledge (understanding and wisdom), and life experiences have been placed between *antecedents* and *critical attributes*. It was the group's decision that these elements were not antecedents, per se, but rather potential enablers, each serving as an impetus for the development of spiritual perspective.

The following conceptual definitions were derived for each concept from the discussions leading to identification of the critical attributes: *spiritual perspective*—an integrating and creative energy based on belief in, and a feeling of interconnectedness with, a power greater than self; *hope*—an energized mental state involving feelings of uneasiness or uncertainty and characterized by a cognitive, action-oriented expectation that a positive future goal or outcome is possible; *acceptance*—a present-oriented activity requiring energy and characterized by receptivity toward and satisfaction with someone or something, including past circumstances, present situations, others, and ultimately, the self; and *self-transcendence*—the experience of extending oneself inwardly in introspective activities, outwardly through concerns about the welfare of others, and temporally, such that the perceptions of one's past and anticipated future enhance the present (Reed, 1991). It is interesting to note that, after a great deal of discussion and analysis, the group adopted Reed's (1991) definition of self-transcendence, providing theoretical validation for her work with this concept. The results of the clarification of individual concepts, including antecedents, critical attributes, and outcomes can be discerned by each concept horizontally across Figure 11–2. Again, do not pay too much attention to the arrows, boxes, and bold type yet.

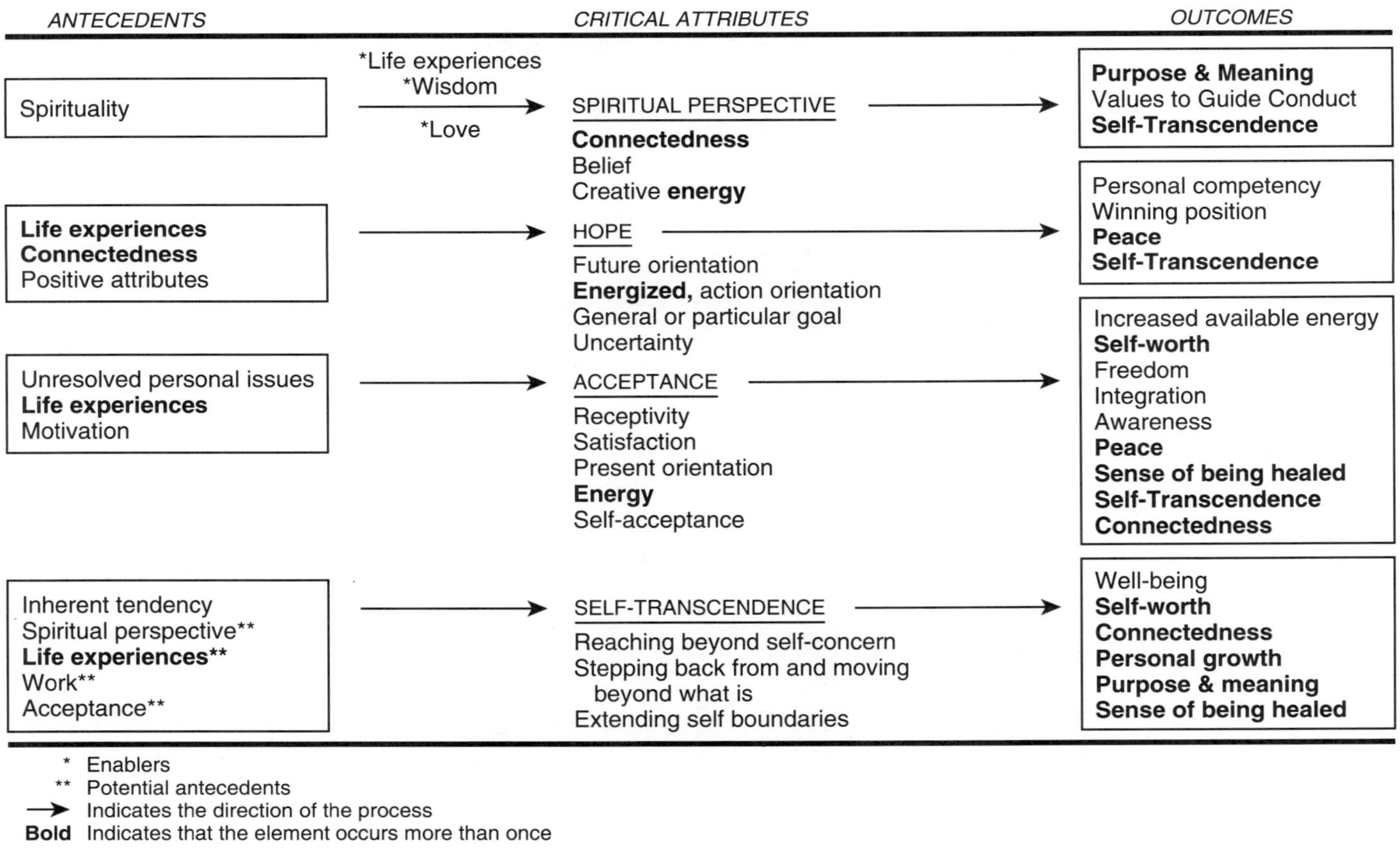

Figure 11–2 Four-concept process model.

ANTECEDENTS   CRITICAL ATTRIBUTES   OUTCOMES

Spirituality

*Life experiences
*Wisdom
*Love

SPIRITUAL PERSPECTIVE
Connectedness
Belief
Creative **energy**

Purpose & Meaning
Values to Guide Conduct
Self-Transcendence

Life experiences
Connectedness
Positive attributes

HOPE
Future orientation
Energized, action orientation
General or particular goal
Uncertainty

Personal competency
Winning position
Peace
Self-Transcendence

Unresolved personal issues
Life experiences
Motivation

ACCEPTANCE
Receptivity
Satisfaction
Present orientation
Energy
Self-acceptance

Increased available energy
Self-worth
Freedom
Integration
Awareness
Peace
Sense of being healed
Self-Transcendence
Connectedness

Inherent tendency
Spiritual perspective**
Life experiences
Work**
Acceptance**

SELF-TRANSCENDENCE
Reaching beyond self-concern
Stepping back from and moving
    beyond what is
Extending self boundaries

Well-being
Self-worth
Connectedness
Personal growth
Purpose & meaning
Sense of being healed

*   Enablers
**   Potential antecedents
→   Indicates the direction of the process
Bold Indicates that the element occurs more than once

183

Group Process Outcomes. Several group process outcomes also resulted from this phase. After several months of meeting, group members felt more comfortable implementing concept clarification techniques in a group setting. In addition, mutual understanding of the four concepts increased. That is, group members felt they had a basic understanding of the structure of all concepts and the theoretical and empirical work that had been done in the area. Eventually, we found that all members were so familiar with each concept that when one member questioned the "identified expert," a third member was able to provide case examples or literature references to answer the question.

Development of Validity Matrices. The next major step in simultaneous concept analysis is the identification of similarities and differences across concepts. In reality, steps 4 and 5 begin to intertwine with time. As individual concepts develop, comparing and contrasting should enter the discussion, as indicated earlier. This is an essential component of SCA, and is, in fact, one of its unique characteristics. Unlike individual concept analysis, where a concept can be developed in isolation, each concept in SCA is developed in light of all others. The comparing and contrasting process helps to refine definitions and clarify antecedents, outcomes, and critical attributes. As these elements are developed, however, a more formal means of cross-concept comparison is needed. This formal mechanism is called a validity matrix.

Description of Validity Matrices. To explore the interrelationships between concepts and achieve theoretical cogency, validity matrices are developed for antecedents, critical attributes, and outcomes. A validity matrix is a tool we developed to identify and display commonalities across concepts; in factor analytic terms, the matrix is used to "extract common factors." An example of a validity matrix for critical attributes is given in Table 11–1. To develop the matrix, concept labels are placed along the horizontal axis and elements assigned to the concepts are listed below their respective labels. Elements that seem to be common across concepts are grouped together. These common elements are given a "common factor" label that is placed along the vertical axis of the matrix. This process is iterative until all the elements are identified within the context of a common factor. The formation of validity matrices forces the group to consider each element in light of all others, comparing and contrasting to identify inconsistencies and gaps and making revisions when appropriate.

In development of the validity matrix for critical attributes (Table 11–1), five factors were identified that were common across the four concepts: time orientation, energy, feeling, and extrapersonal and intrapersonal orientation. Interestingly, these "common factors" were also used as a means of differentiating the four concepts. For example, three of the concepts

Table 11–1 *Validity Matrix for Critical Attributes*

FACTOR	SPIRITUAL PERSPECTIVE	HOPE	ACCEPTANCE	SELF-TRANSCENDENCE
Time orientation	——	Future	Present	Across time
Energy	Creative	Action	Nonspecific	Derived
Feeling	Connectedness	Uncertainty	Satisfaction	——
Extrapersonal orientation	Belief Connectedness with others/universe	Goal toward others	Receptivity to others	Reaching out
Intrapersonal orientation	Connectedness with self	Goal toward self	Receptivity to self	Extends self boundaries inwardly

were found to be characterized by some form of time orientation, a commonality. However, the concepts could be differentiated from one another by the nature of this time orientation, that is, future, present, or across time, respectively. Similarly, although energy was a common theme across all concepts, the four could be differentiated by the type of energy involved: creative, action, nonspecific, and derived from other sources (perhaps from hope or acceptance).

While we found that some factors assisted us in identifying distinguishing characteristics across concepts, other factors helped us to identify commonalities and potential sources of confusion across concepts. For example, in the validity matrix for outcomes, we found that all four concepts had either connectedness, purpose and meaning, or self-transcendence as common outcome elements. There were no higher order factor labels for them. That is, we were unable to reduce these characteristics to a common denominator; they were irreducible and contributed in this manner to the meaning of each concept. In addition, self-transcendence was itself an outcome element of all other concepts. Thus, research exploring the outcomes of spiritual perspective, hope, and acceptance may reveal repeating themes that may be, and very likely are, characteristics of self-transcendence. (In the interest of available space, all validity matrices are not reproduced here. The reader is referred to Haase et al. [1992] for a more detailed presentation of these SCA findings.)

The validity matrix also allowed us to examine elements within concepts across factors. For example, in Table 11−1 the goal-directed behavior that characterized hope "loaded" on two factors, extrapersonal and intrapersonal orientation. This highlights the proposition that hope-oriented goals can have different referents, either self or others but not necessarily both.

Revision of Individual Concept Clarifications. The construction of validity matrices is designed to help the group critically evaluate the clarity of the identified antecedents, attributes, and outcomes, and the interrelationships and differences that exist across concepts. It is also intended to point out any glaring omissions or inconsistencies in the work accomplished to this point. Logically, the next step in the SCA process is to reexamine the previous concept clarifications and make any necessary revisions. Steps 5 and 6 are clearly interrelated and iterative processes.

For example, our original work on the concept of acceptance did not include receptivity as a critical attribute. When we constructed the matrix and initially found no element for acceptance that fit extrapersonal or intrapersonal orientation, we began to question whether we had overlooked a critical attribute of acceptance. We identified receptivity to self and others as a critical attribute. Although receptivity seems an obvious component of acceptance now, it may not have been realized had it not been for the use of SCA and validity matrices.

Reexamination of Validity Matrices. Once again, the iterative nature of the SCA process is apparent. Group discussion, examination, and reexamination of the concept analyses and validity matrices are essential to the development of multiple concepts.

Our experiences with the development of the validity matrix method and its subsequent use have led to several precautions: First, as indicated, there is a danger of trying to force-fit elements into a common factor. In reexamination and review it is imperative that the group avoid the temptation to overmassage, to the point that insignificant characteristics are included that contribute little to the understanding of the concepts or their underlying processes. In analyzing the four concepts discussed here, some commonalities among elements were relatively easy to identify and label. Others were more difficult to reconcile. Perhaps the best words of advice: if it ain't broke, don't fix it—change only that which really needs to be changed.

Second, careful consideration should be given to semantics and terminology. This is particularly important in exercises such as this, where language—that is, communication—is the central issue. For example, in the validity matrix for outcomes we held lengthy discussions about the difference in meaning between the common factor label, serenity, and an outcome, peace. Through this discusssion and a timely meeting with Kay Roberts concerning her qualitative studies of serenity (Roberts & Fitzgerald, 1991), we were able to come to some agreement.

Development of a Process Model. As the definitions, antecedents, outcomes, and attributes become more clearly delineated, the need for a process model evolves. A process model is a structure to further examine the consistency and pattern among concepts under analysis. In many respects it is a reflection of Kaplan's (1964) description of models as "devices by which a system can be shown to be consistent" (p. 267) and that offer "meaningful contexts within which specific findings can be located as significant details" (p. 268). It is a grand overview, a single image of the elements and processes of the analyzed concepts in juxtaposition. In one apparently complex, but meaningful picture, the group is able to examine each concept, the similarities and differences across concepts, the interrelationships across both concepts and processes, and new concepts that appear in strategic locations throughout the model. A process model is not intended, in any way, to represent theory. Rather, it should be seen as an analytic tool and a predecessor of theory.

Figure 11−2 is a process model of the four concepts we analyzed using the SCA strategy. Examples of a few of the insights gained through this model are as follows. Note that spiritual perspective, characterized by connectedness, belief, and creative energy, was found to be an antecedent of self-transcendence. This implies that life experiences, wisdom, and love as enablers of spiritual perspective, might contribute to self-transcendence indirectly, through their impact on the development of self-transcendence. Purpose and meaning are outcomes of spiritual perspective and self-transcendence, indicating there are several paths to the evolution of these two outcomes. Note, too, that life experiences are antecedents of all concepts. This is consistent with the notion that personal growth and the development of personal resources of spiritual perspective, hope, acceptance, and self-transcendence, arise out of life experiences.

Another theme that became apparent through Figure 11–2 is the central role of intrapersonal characteristics for each of these concepts. That is, wisdom and love are enablers of spiritual perspective, positive attributes such as optimism are antecedents of hope, motivation is an antecedent of acceptance, and spiritual perspective and acceptance are antecedents of self-transcendence. Intrapersonal characteristics appear as critical attributes as well, and include, for example, connectedness with self, receptivity, and extended self boundaries. Many outcomes also reflected the intrapersonal characteristics theme, including such personal growth characteristics as the development of personal values, competency, self-worth and well-being.

Finally, an important *new* concept emerged as a central theme: connectedness. Connectedness with others is an antecedent of hope, a critical attribute of spiritual perspective, and a consequence of acceptance and self-transcendence. This suggests that the apparent theoretical overlap among the four concepts may also be due, in part, to a connectedness that crosses all four psychosocial phenomena. In some sense, this finding was not surprising, nor, of course, is the concept really new. Burkhardt's (1989) concept analysis proposed harmonious interconnectedness as the central characteristic of spirituality, and, intuitively, a sense of connectedness with others should be an important part of each of these concepts. Yet, the centrality of connectedness to all four concepts was made apparent to us through the SCA strategy. Furthermore, since the four concepts were selected because of their perceived importance to nursing, the implications of connectedness for the nursing profession seem even more meaningful and dynamic.

Submission of the SCA Results to Peers for Critique. The final step in the SCA process is to submit the findings to one or more peers for review. After they have worked closely with many complex concepts, it is easy for the researchers to lose perspective. Thus, it is helpful to seek objective evaluation of the results. Do they seem logical? Are the terms consistent across concepts? What are the implications of the findings for theory development and research? Do the findings have potential meaning for nursing practice?

By presenting the results informally to peers, to colleagues in seminar, or to refereed journals for broader review, the SCA process can come full circle, presenting opportunities for reworking the same concepts, or moving on to new ones. Connectedness, for example, awaits further analyses by an enthusiastic SCA team.

IMPLICATIONS

What Can SCA Tell Us about Empirical Methods? It is interesting that implications concerning qualitative and quantitative empirical methods arise from the simultaneous clarification process. Qualitative implications include the need for *field studies* to further clarify the concepts of interest, as well as those emerging from the SCA strategy. Among the quantitative implications are issues related to measurement, model specification, the use of latent variables, and assumptions underlying commonly used statistical methods. In addition, SCA can provide guidance for programs of research, suggesting empirical work to explore, verify, or test SCA findings.

Schwartz-Barcott and Kim (1986), in their hybrid model for concept development, suggested that investigators and theorists use field research methods to empirically validate a concept. Such qualitative data would contribute to the clarity and validity of concept analyses obtained through SCA, and could be a useful component of this strategy. On the other hand, qualitative studies conducted by individual group members could be a useful goal or outcome as well. In fact, phenomenological studies would be useful predecessors of SCA to obtain an understanding of the structure of the concept, whereas ethnographic or grounded theory approaches could contribute to clarifying the social and cultural processes associated with the model (Morse, 1991).

In terms of quantitative measurement issues, confirmational factor analyses of instruments designed to measure multidimensional concepts should be performed in order to evaluate factor structures in light of the definitions, interrelationships, and validity matrices proposed through SCA. Because multidimensional concepts, such as those presented in this chapter, often represent changing processes, investigators should anticipate low to moderate test-retest reliability in their instruments, particularly during times of pivotal life events or experiences. In selecting or developing instruments to measure multidimensional and interrelated concepts, consideration must be given to the nature of their interrelationships and the goal of the study or program of research. If a critical goal is to differentiate among any combination of the variables, for example, the instruments should be restricted to critical attributes, the area least likely to contain overlap. On the other hand, if the goal is to measure outcomes, the investigator must remain aware of the similarities and differences obtained in SCA, and how these are reflected in the various instruments. High correlations among the outcomes of spiritual perspective, hope, acceptance, and self-transcendence would be expected due to their similarities along this dimension. To gain more accurate insight into the interrelationships among outcomes of these four variables, the researcher might consider restricting measurement to one unique outcome for each concept, rather than attempting to tap all dimensions.

Concepts amenable to SCA often involve dynamic and interrelated processes. Hence, they are likely to be excellent candidates for latent variable and nonrecursive models. Latent variable modeling, a statistical procedure that uses multiple indicators to measure a single factor, would enable the investigator to account for the shared and unique variances of both instruments and latent factors. Nonrecursive modeling, a statistical procedure that can accommodate feedback loops, is the appropriate technique for examining the various reoccurring processes that may be suggested by simultaneous concept analysis. Process models may be used as an initial step in the development of theoretical models to be subjected to empirical testing.

Clearly, the study of interrelated concepts can create numerous analytical problems. SCA may assist the investigator in anticipating and visualizing some of these. For example, simple regression analysis is designed to handle a certain degree of multicollinearity, the intercorrelation among the independent variables. When multicollinearity is extreme, however, problems arise, specifically large standard errors of estimation and failure to achieve statistical significance. This, of course, makes it difficult to obtain a unique solution for the parameter estimates; that is, it becomes difficult to separate out the effects of the interrelated variables, often the task of greatest interest (see Berry & Feldman, 1985; Lewis-Beck, 1980; or Pedhazur, 1982 for more complete discussions of multicollinearity). SCA should provide the investigator with some insight into the potential for multicollinearity; especially its source and potential solutions. For example, the degree of overlap among outcomes of the four concepts considered here suggests that unless special precautions are taken, a high degree of multicollinearity would be inevitable. Hence, these four concepts do not appear to be good candidates for the role of independent variables in a simple regression model.

Finally, implications for specific empirical work should arise from the SCA process. For example, life experiences, connectedness, and positive attributes were found to be antecedents of hope in our SCA. The qualitative and quantitative research implications of this statement are important. What is connectedness? How is it experienced? What are positive attributes? How do these characteristics differ for people experiencing hope (according to the critical attributes identified) and those who are not? Is self-transcendence an outcome of hope? In what way are hope and self-transcendence helpful to clients of nursing? In what way can (do) nurses facilitate hope through connectedness? Are there specific interventions that can be tested? The ideas that arise from SCA can be endless.

What Does SCA Tell Us about the Philosophical Aspects of Concept Development in Nursing? It is difficult to say whether SCA has inherent philosophical implications, or if the method reflects the philosophical bases of the group developing the strategy. In any event, there are philosophical underpinnings to the SCA approach, and it is to these that we must now turn before discussion of this strategy can be considered complete.

Several philosophical assumptions clearly underlie the SCA strategy. First and foremost, concepts relevant to nursing are viewed as complex, interrelated, dynamic processes. Thus, to consider or analyze them as static terms provides a false understanding of their underlying structure or processes. Second, because such interrelationships exist, many concepts cannot, and should not, be analyzed in isolation. The influence of related concepts can significantly alter the dynamic processes that occur. Hence the development of the SCA strategy. Third, to obtain a holistic product, concept analyses should reflect diverse perspectives. And, to the extent possible, results should be useful to theorists, investigators, and practitioners in a variety of settings. This is the most useful contribution concept analysis can make to the language of nursing and its development as a discipline. Finally, qualitative and quantitative research have important, complementary, noncompeting roles in nursing science. Together, these methodologies can provide a scientific data base for nursing practice and further the development of nursing theory.

UNANSWERED QUESTIONS

Although we found the SCA strategy to be effective in deriving greater understanding and insight concerning concepts of interest to us, others must use and evaluate the method in order to prove its utility. Because it is offered as a new, alternative approach to concept analysis there are, of course, a number of unanswered questions. For example, is SCA feasible without a consensus group? That is, is it possible for one individual to "objectively" conduct an SCA? To "master" more than one concept without group challenge? At this point, we think it is not. The group consensus process is an integral part, and strength, of SCA. To attempt simultaneous analyses alone would yield different, and perhaps less interesting, results due to the loss of varied perspective offered by the group approach.

A second question concerns the laying aside of interesting and rich subtleties of individual concepts in an attempt to handle large quantities of information more efficiently and gain breadth of understanding across concepts. This problem was introduced in the discussion of step 4. At this point, a question remains as to what to do with these rich subtleties. What, if anything, was lost here? Did the gain in breadth offset any loss in depth? Should the group return to earlier steps in the SCA process and reevaluate each concept, integrating the information that was set aside? Or should this task be left to individuals during their research pursuits? Can further individual analyses be done without threatening the validity of findings from SCAs? We hope that groups using the SCA will revisit some of their earlier work and evaluate the extent to which information was lost and can be reintegrated into the SCA results. Not all groups will have this opportunity, however. In these situations, it is likely, and desirable, that individuals return to their independent projects with greater insight into their own, and related concepts. Further independent concept clarification may prove useful. SCA is designed to be one of many strategies used to clarify concepts and strengthen professional language. It should complement other approaches and withstand the test offered by subjecting the results to further concept clarification.

SUMMARY

Simultaneous concept analysis (SCA) is a strategy designed to generate and refine conceptual definitions, critical attributes, theoretical definitions, antecedents, and outcomes of multiple interrelated concepts. Critical components of this strategy are consensus group process, the application of validity matrices, and the development of a process model. Unlike the individual concept analysis approach proposed by Wilson (1969), and Walker and Avant (1988), the SCA strategy is designed to analyze interrelationships and identify theoretical overlap, common themes, and distinguishing characteristics among similar or complementary concepts. It is a new strategy that must be subjected to further scrutiny and evaluation. Nevertheless, the method proved very useful to us in clarifying four complex, interrelated, and empirically elusive concepts. We hope that it will prove useful for others as well.

REFERENCES

Berry, W., & Feldman, S. (1985). *Multiple regression in practice.* Beverly Hills: Sage.

Burkhardt, M. (1989). Spirituality: An analysis of the concept. *Holistic Nursing Practice, 3*(3), 69–77.

Haase, J., Britt, T., Coward, D., Kline Leidy, N., & Penn, P. (1992). Simultaneous concept analysis of spiritual perspective, hope, acceptance, and self-transcendence. *Image, 24,* 141–147.

Kaplan, A. (1964). *The conduct of inquiry.* Philadelphia: Chandler.

Lewis-Beck (1980). *Applied regression: An introduction.* Beverly Hills: Sage.

Morse, J.M. (1991). *Qualitative nursing research: A contemporary dialogue* (rev. ed.). Newbury Park, Calif: Sage.

Pedhazur, E. (1982). *Multiple regression in behavioral research: Explanation and prediction* (2nd ed). New York: Holt, Rinehart, & Winston.

Reed, P. (1991). Self-transcendence and mental health in oldest-old adults. *Nursing Research, 40,* 5–11.

Roberts, K., & Fitzgerald, L. (1991). Serenity: Caring with perspective. *Scholarly Inquiry for Nursing Practice, 5*(2), 127–142.

Schwartz-Barcott, D., & Kim, H. S. (1986). A hybrid model for concept development. In P. Chinn (Ed.), *Nursing research: Methodology issues and instrumentation.* Rockville, Md: Aspen.

Walker, L., & Avant, K. (1988). *Strategies for theory construction in nursing* (2nd ed.). Norwalk, Conn: Appleton & Lange.

Wilson, J. (1969). *Thinking with concepts.* New York: Cambridge University Press.

Chapter 12

Integrative Literature Reviews in the Development of Concepts

MARION E. BROOME

*A*ny individual who chooses to systematically build a base of knowledge about a selected concept will be involved in searching, reading, analyzing, and eventually reconceptualizing existing literature on the concept. Interestingly, searching the literature is one of the earliest skills required in education, yet one most often taken for granted. Little attention is given to teaching the students the skills required to conduct a thorough literature search, critique the research, and report their findings. Instead, most students develop a routine approach to selecting and reviewing the literature and consistently follow this routine without regard to its effectiveness.

The volumes of information published daily on any given topic have become overwhelming (Cooper, 1989). It is estimated that the average scholar spends eight to ten hours a week reading, and that he or she consistently scans seven journals in a selected area of interest and follows four others on a regular basis (*Scholarly Communication,* 1979). Obviously, anyone beginning the study of a concept must use a systematic and thorough method to search and analyze the literature in order to minimize effort and maximize knowledge gained.

The primary purpose of a review of the literature is to gain an in-depth understanding of a phenomenon by building on the work of others. This process is especially important in concept development. Concept building requires a working knowledge of what previous work has been done in the area as well as what questions remain unanswered. Such a review will assist the individual to develop a personal definition of the concept, to understand how others have measured related phenomena, and to identify the various dimensions of the concept. It is essential that the sources that are chosen are as representative of the entire body of literature as possible. This is especially important when the reader is interested in broadening knowledge about a concept. How the investigator organizes the search, how the content of the literature is documented, what methods are used to critically analyze each piece of the literature, and finally, how the content is organized, synthesized, and presented can be very time consuming. In some cases this work becomes unproductive, especially if the entire process lacks organization and direction.

Rigorous, systematic reviews of the literature are critical to developing a substantial knowledge base about a concept. Approaches to learning and eventually to contributing knowledge about a concept should be as uncompromising as any other step in the knowledge building and testing process. The purpose of this chapter is to discuss methods that are used by researchers to systematically search and analyze the literature as well as strategies that investigators use to critically evaluate sources and organize and synthesize their findings.

Types of Literature Reviews

There are several types of reviews commonly seen in journals, books, or manuscripts. These vary in purpose, scope, depth, breadth, and organization of the material. Reviews include abbreviated synopses of the literature found in most data-based research articles, methodological reviews, theoretical reviews, critical reviews, integrative reviews, and meta-analyses. These various approaches share some commonalities, yet have divergent goals. For instance, a theoretical review of pediatric pain (Beyer & Byers, 1985) includes some of the same research used in a meta-analysis of pediatric pain management strategies (Broome, Lillis, & Smith, 1989). The purpose of the first, a theoretical review, is much broader and inclusive of the literature evaluated and discussed. Theoretical reviews often include a historical analysis of the "state of the science" and recommendations for further theory development and research in the area. The primary purpose of a meta-analysis is to examine the overall effectiveness of specific interventions, in this case pain management, and is more focused on a review of selected intervention studies.

Abbreviated Reviews. Abbreviated reviews found in journal articles are typically much shorter than other types, due to space limitations. These reviews are narrowly focused around a discussion of the variables and empirical data in that specific study. A limitation of such reviews is the limited scope and selective nature of what is presented; usually only research that is supportive to the argument for the present research is included.

Methodological Reviews. A methodological review is focused on critiquing the designs, methods, and analyses in a series of studies. An example of such a review is Fullerton and Wingard's (1990) "Methodological Problems in the Assessment of Nurse-Midwifery Practice." These authors reviewed the research conducted over 30 years and discussed the process, structure, and outcomes of these studies. Limitations of the studies were described and specific suggestions for further research were provided.

Theoretical Reviews. A theoretical review is perhaps the most challenging to write and yet can be very instrumental in moving collective thought ahead in a discipline. These reviews usually propose models that describe the relationships among variables previously studied, and often propose new variables and relationships to investigate. Hence, they tend to be most useful for and relevant to concept development. Occasionally, these reviews result in the identification and description of a new concept or theory. An example is Thompson's (1990) discussion of the concept of "developmental venerability" of children participating in research.

Critical Reviews. Critical reviews are extensive analyses of literature in a selected area that usually have a specific focus. Such reviews do not include original data but rather are interpretations of findings from different studies. A specific concept (e.g., day care) is defined, and a concise historical perspective on the topic is provided. Critical reviews are comprehensive and include both a theoretical analysis and methodological critique of the research. Most authors use this synthesis of the literature to develop theoretical propositions that generate many fruitful ideas for future research. An excellent example of a comprehensive, critical review article is "Supporting Families During Chronic Illness" (Woods, Yates, & Primomo, 1989) in which the concepts of chronic illness, demands of illness, and social support are discussed. The authors reviewed empirical data in those areas, discussed the relationships between nurses' support and chronic illness and identified several testable propositions.

Integrative Reviews. An integrative review is defined as one in which past research is summarized by drawing overall conclusions from many studies. Although this is very similar to the kind of work done and presented in a critical review, there are some distinct differences. Cooper (1989) recommended formulating a research problem that will guide the integrative review. He defined *research problem* broadly, and stressed that definitions of important variables and a description of how the variables relate to one another should be included. This first step of identifying the research problem or question is important in order to delimit the scope of the review. For instance, even in a topic area with a relatively recent research history, such as neonatal pain, much has been written. This literature varies a great deal and includes studies of behavioral responses of the neonate to painful procedures as well as comparative studies of pharmacologic options such as fentanyl and morphine.

A question or hypothesis such as "Is morphine or fentanyl more effective in reducing pain in the neonate?" or a broader question such as "Which analgesics are most effective in reducing neonatal pain?" is very effective in delimiting the review. Although this second question broadens the scope of the review it still restricts the type of literature to that reporting pharmacologic interventions and would exclude studies in which the primary purpose was to examine behavioral responses to neonatal pain.

Meta-Analysis. Meta-analysis is a special case of the integrative review. The purpose of meta-analysis is to conduct an integrative review and, in addition, to determine the overall effectiveness of interventions. In a meta-analysis, selected variables related to research or the phenomenon itself are examined to determine their influence on an intervention's effectiveness.

Questions that Guide Review Processes. As any student or scholar knows, there is much to be gained from reading a variety of reviews on a selected topic. For individuals interested in concept development, these reviews are invaluable and facilitate mastery of a broad literature. During the review process answers to the following questions should be sought:

1. How has the concept been defined by authors and what is the range of experiences of the concept?
2. What factors and variables are significant in a given area? (Tuckman, 1978; Woods, 1988)
3. What work has already been done and what can be expanded? (Cooper, 1989; Tuckman, 1978; Woods, 1988)
4. What relationships have been discovered between dimensions of this concept and other related phenomena? (Tuckman, 1978; Woods, 1988)
5. What theoretical perspectives and research traditions have been used to understand the concept?

Integrative Reviews and Meta-Analyses

There have been several attempts by nursing authors to direct attention to the need for a more systematic and rigorous approach to the review of the literature. Ganong (1987) critiqued 17 integrative reviews in nursing published from 1978 to 1983 in four major research journals. One meta-analysis was included in this sample. Ganong found that only 9 of the 17 reviews included discussion of methodological problems, while 3 presented a systematic search for effects. All but 1 review provided suggestions for further research, and 6 reviews discussed implications for policy or practice. Only 1 review included suggestions for further research. Ganong concluded that although methods for conducting integrative reviews vary, they should be as uncompromising as methods for conducting primary research and a systematic, thoughtful process should be used in reviewing the literature. That process is discussed in the rest of this chapter. Meta-analysis, which is a unique, extended form of the integrative review, has received a great deal of attention in most practice disciplines. Nursing is no exception, so a discussion of meta-analysis is included. The processes of conducting integrative reviews and meta-analyses share many commonalities, as shown in Table 12–1. Meta-analysis takes the integrative review one step further, reanalyzes the data reported in each article, and determines the overall effectiveness of a specific research treatment.

CONCEPT IDENTIFICATION AND RESEARCH QUESTIONS

The broader the scope of the chosen concept, the more selective the integrative reviewer will have to be about the literature used. For instance, if one chooses to study the experience of an adolescent's response to situational stresses, one could identify several concepts that would vary in their breadth and depth, such as stress, coping, and maturation.

Once the concept is chosen, questions that will guide the review are identified to delimit the search and facilitate identification of the key words (Smith, 1987). Specifically, the questions that guide the review or meta-

Table 12–1   *Process of Integrative Reviews and Meta-Analysis*

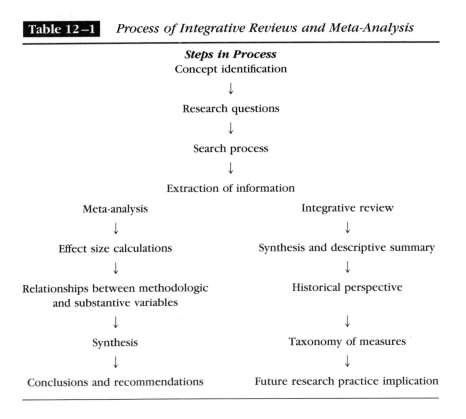

	Steps in Process	
	Concept identification	
	↓	
	Research questions	
	↓	
	Search process	
	↓	
	Extraction of information	
Meta-analysis		**Integrative review**
↓		↓
Effect size calculations		Synthesis and descriptive summary
↓		↓
Relationships between methodologic and substantive variables		Historical perspective
↓		↓
Synthesis		Taxonomy of measures
↓		↓
Conclusions and recommendations		Future research practice implication

analysis should be made explicit because they will influence which studies are chosen, what information is extracted from the articles, and which statistical operations, if any, are chosen to analyze the data. The research questions for reviews can be broad or narrow; however, broad questions make the review very labor intensive.

The research questions will be a reflection of the theoretical perspective and underlying assumptions held by the investigator, and can heavily influence the interpretation of the findings (Smith, 1987). For instance, in two different meta-analyses of the pain literature (Broome, Lillis, & Smith, 1989; Fernandez & Turk, 1989), different categorizations of cognitive coping strategies were used. Broome, Lillis, and Smith restricted their meta-analysis to research interventions with children and reported types of interventions (cognitive, biophysical, and affective), while Fernandez and Turk restricted their review to cognitive strategies only, using studies with primarily adult subjects. Both groups of researchers reported that cognitive strategies were beneficial in reducing pain and distress ratings. The intervention categories in Fernandez and Turk's paper were more discrete, which reflected the purpose of the paper as well as the background and interests of the authors, who were psychologists.

Once the research questions are specified, decision making related to the sample of studies to be reviewed begins. For instance, the reviewer has to decide if the literature search will be restricted to one or several disciplines and how many years will be searched. These decisions are heavily influenced by the historical evolution of the concept itself as well as how discipline specific a concept is. For instance, the concept of maternal confidence is prevalent in the nursing literature, nonexistent in medicine, and labeled self-efficacy in psychology. Some of these decisions are arbitrary, and different investigators will choose different options to guide their search.

THE SEARCH PROCESS

There are a variety of ways to locate sources. Newer search technologies are always evolving, and the reviewer should always talk with reference librarians in order to identify which new additions are most useful.

Most research texts contain a comprehensive list and descriptions of the various computerized literature searches (Burns & Grove 1987; Tuckman 1978; Wilson, 1985; Woods, 1988). There is a certain degree of skill and knowledge required to conduct a computerized search and anyone who is seriously considering conducting one should spend time in the library either with a reference librarian, a tutorial specific to literature searches, or in a library sponsored class. In the long run, much time will be saved and the outcomes of the search will be maximized.

If the literature to be searched is very extensive, the use of questions that can guide the review is critical. These questions will also help the reviewer to later identify key words to delimit the search. For instance, the concept of *pain* is extremely broad and will yield 43,330 citations on MEDLINE from 1966 to 1983. Some narrowing is necessary in order to conduct a timely, efficient but thorough search. The following questions are examples of how such a broad topic could be narrowed:

1. When was pain first identified in the cancer literature? What kinds of pain do cancer patients have?
2. How is pain measured in cancer patients?
3. What are the common modalities used to test cancer pain?

Obvious key words in a search of literature to answer these questions are *cancer, pain, measurement,* and *intervention.* However, it is possible that very little would emerge from an initial search using just those key words especially to answer question 3. The reviewer may need to search a broader literature on pain assessment using computerized on-line search procedures such as MEDLINE and CANCERLINE (see Table 12–2). To use these most efficiently, the reviewer must continue to identify *key words* that will assist the individual conducting the search and narrow the field.

For instance, a search that begins with a global concept such as *pain* is narrowed considerably by the descriptor *pediatric pain* and even further with *pediatric pain assessment.* Additional key words that could be used to narrow the search for articles reporting research in pediatric pain assessment may be *child response, pain measurement,* and *procedural pain.*

In most libraries, anyone can search a number of data bases at no charge using the mini-MEDLINE on a library information system. Other searches that are more comprehensive require the use of personnel and computer time and may be costly. Each data base charges a different amount depending on the number of citations retrieved, the computer time used, and the extent of the entire literature base.

An alternative to the computerized search, but one I find works well, is to initially use article bibliographies, or reference lists from very recent books on the subject. This is a rather commonly used approach called the descendency method (Cooper, 1987). A study of 57 authors of research reviews published in psychology and education revealed the use of references in published review papers to be the most frequently reported strategy for searching the literature. In addition, authors stated they often communicated with others who shared their work or ideas, a concept commonly referred to as "the invisible college" (Crane, 1969). Computer searches of abstract data bases, such as ERIC or Psychological Abstracts, were also used. Least commonly reported strategies were government agency lists, computer searches of citation indexes, and browsing through the library.

Even in searches limited by time, resources, and money, the goal should be to avoid obvious bias in a search within the limits of cost (Cooper, 1989). It is important to not overrepresent any one segment of the literature and thereby reduce generalizability of the conclusions. Yet, cost of retrieval,

Table 12-2 Computer Search Services

HEALTH SCIENCES

AIDSLINE is a new and dynamic database on the acquired immunodeficiency syndrome. Available from the National Library of Medicine.

BIOSIS contains citations from both Biological Abstracts and Biological Abstracts/RRM. Research literature in the life sciences is comprehensively covered through the abstracting of articles from 9,000+ journals, congresses, reviews, reports, and research communication.

CANCERLINE (sponsored by the National Cancer Institute) contains citations and abstracts from journals, congresses, conferences, and texts. All aspects of cancer are covered including radio-, chemo-, and immuno-therapies, radiation injuries, and carcinogenesis.

MEDLINE produced by the National Library of Medicine, corresponds to three printed indexes: Index Medicus, International Nursing Index, and Index to Dental Literature. Indexing articles from 3,200+ journals published in over 70 countries, it is a major source of biomedical information.

NURSING & ALLIED HEALTH LITERATURE (CINAHL) contains citations to English language journal articles and some pamphlet and other ephemeral materials in the disciplines of nursing, medical technology, physical therapy, and other allied health science professions.

BIOETHICSLINE includes interdisciplinary coverage of bioethical topics such as euthanasia, abortion, biotechnology. Information is compiled from a variety of formats: books, journals, newspapers, court cases, and audio-visuals.

Psych INFO produced by the American Psychological Association, contains references and abstracts to the literature of psychology and related disciplines. The formats of the indexed literature include periodicals, dissertations, technical reports, and conference proceedings.

SOCIAL SCISEARCH is a multidisciplinary database indexing 100 primary journals in the social sciences, and selected articles from 2,000+ additional journals from other fields. The unique feature of this data base is the capability of producing lists of current references that have cited a well-known paper or author.

breadth of the literature, specificity of the research questions, and time restrictions all influence how extensive the search will be. When decisions are made about the search process they should be documented, and the search must reflect these decisions. For instance, in the meta-analysis by Broome, Lillis, and Smith (1989), a decision was made to begin the search with 1967 and extend over the next 20 years through December, 1987. The beginning date was chosen because it was 10 years before the first systematic studies of pediatric pain emerged. To increase comprehensiveness and include literature from several disciplines, these authors scanned an index of health profession journals that listed 1,000 journals. Journals that were chosen from this index were those thought to include pediatric pain intervention studies. All of these decisions and procedures were documented, and the records were kept in a notebook. This documentation was very useful two years later when the meta-analysis was being presented and written up for publication.

Searches often proceed in levels that begin broad and increasingly narrow. Searching the literature is never strictly a linear process but rather one in which the author returns many times to the initial questions and decision criteria when choosing what to do next. Initially, as was discussed earlier, key words are developed to assist in screening the studies. During the meta-analysis discussed earlier, Broome, Lillis, and Smith (1989) identified 32 key words such as *pain, interventions,* and *child,* for a computerized search using MEDLINE and dissertation abstracts. This Level I search yielded 125 articles and dissertations on pain interventions with children. Many of these were descriptive studies or clinical case studies. In a second level of review, it was decided that the research study must report use of an intervention, include more than 10 subjects, and contain the statistical information necessary to calculate effect sizes. These criteria were based on both initial research questions and meta-analysis methodology. In this particular meta-analysis, the statistical procedures used to determine effect size required information about the number of subjects, the type of statistical tests run, and statistical values (e.g., n = 119; statistic = t-test and value = 2.43).

A total of 27 studies were finally included in the meta-analysis. Nonpublished studies and unpublished theses were not included because the investigators decided that using only published material and dissertations would provide assurance of a minimal quality of the study. Their assumption was based on the belief that journal referees and university dissertation committee members provide some consistency in the quality of written research reports. Time limitations and cost constraints on this meta-analysis also influenced this decision. If masters theses and solicitation of unpublished studies are used the search process is extended considerably. This decision is an example of one of the decisions that can differ depending on the reviewer, as others might choose to invest more time and money to include a wider range of sources. Again, decisions were documented and studies that were excluded in the meta-analysis were listed in a bibliography with a notation as to the reason for the exclusion. The authors found this documentation very helpful later when responding to questions about why specific articles were not included.

EXTRACTION OF INFORMATION

Annotation of articles from the literature involves the extraction of specific information from an article. The purpose of annotation is to summarize and document, in a concise and easily retrievable way, information from each piece of literature. Important content can vary with each reviewer's purposes but generally includes the purpose, methodology, and findings of the study. Annotation can be done in a variety of ways. Traditionally, index cards have been used by reviewers to organize their assessments of each article. With the increasing popularity of personal computers, many reviewers now use charts to organize relevant content using software programs such as Word Perfect. One advantage to the chart system is that studies can be viewed and compared easily as a whole, as shown in Table 12−3. Although categories in the chart are flexible they should reflect the overall purpose of the review. Organizing the articles chronologically allows the individual to develop an appreciation for the historical evolution of knowledge in the area.

CODING

Coding information taken from the articles is a two-step process. First, the reviewer develops a codebook that guides which information is retrieved from the article. The second step requires an assessment of the quality of the research. Codebooks are used in both integrative reviews and meta-analyses (Cooper, 1989; McCain, Smith, & Abraham, 1986). Selection of what information to extract varies. Investigators must have a working knowledge of the concept as well as methodologies used in the research in order to develop the codebook (Smith, 1987). An example of a section of the codebook used by my colleagues and me for a meta-analysis can be found in Table 12−4. Relevant methodological and substantive variables are listed and applied to each article. Information in the codebook is very important and will be used in later analyses to determine if overall effect sizes were affected by any methodological or substantive variables. For example, the researcher might want to consider whether the type of intervention used, such as distraction or parental presence, was related to children's responses to pain, or whether sampling methods were reflective of sample size.

Developing the codebook and coding the initial studies is a reciprocal process requiring many revisions as it becomes clear that data are missing or not available in the form required (Cooper, 1989). A draft of the code-

Table 12–3 *Chart to Annotate Literature: Studies of Nurses' Pain Medication Practices in Pediatrics*

AUTHOR	YEAR	SAMPLE	DIAGNOSIS	FINDINGS
Eland & Anderson	1977	*Matched Sample*: 25 children 5-8 years old; matched with 18 adults	Postoperative pain	Only 3 of 12 children received narcotics for a total of 24 doses; 18 adults received 372 narcotics and 299 nonnarcotics for a total of 671 doses in same time period.
Beyer, DeGood, Ashley, & Russell	1983	*Random Sample*: 50 children, 50 adults	Postoperative open heart surgery	No pain medications were prescribed for six subjects who were children. Potent narcotics were prescribed and administered significantly less often for children than for adults. Mean of 8.3 versus 3.2 doses administered 3 days postop. Five days postop 21% (6) of children received a total of 10 doses while 96% (48) of adults received total of 136 doses.
Mather & Mackie	1983	Chart review 170 pediatric patients	Postoperative pain	No medication ordered for 16%; narcotics ordered, but not given to 39%. In 30%, nonnarcotic was substituted exclusively for order where narcotic and nonnarcotic

Continued.

Table 12–3   *Chart to Annotate Literature: Studies of Nurses' Pain Medication Practices in Pediatrics*   Continued

AUTHOR	YEAR	SAMPLE	DIAGNOSIS	FINDINGS
				were ordered. *Only 25% of patients were pain free day of surgery;* 13% reported severe pain, although 75% received narcotics.
Burokas	1985	Survey of chart review of 40 charges of pediatric patients	Postoperative pain	Nurses chose to intervene with medication more often than not with variability in choice of strength of dose; 90% reported 1-month-old feels pain.
Gadish	1988	Chart reviews and questionnaires for 68 pediatric nurses on postop unit	Postoperative pain	Nurses identified medication as primary intervention (84%). Almost half also reported using nonmedication interventions. More often they chose nonnarcotic and lower dosage narcotics for younger children; 63% had goal of relieving as much pain as possible; 84% would give pain injection even if child denies pain.

Table 12–4 Selected Examples of Variables in a Codebook

Methodological Characteristics

Journal type (nursing, medicine, dental)	Nursing (1)
Setting (in-patients, clinic, dental office)	Clinic (2)
Sample (infants, toddlers, male, female)	Preschoolers (3) Both genders (3)
Sampling procedures (random selection, convenience)	Random assignment (2)
Size of experimental group; control group	n = 37 n = 36

Substantive

Type of intervention (cognitive, affective, biophysical)	Cognitive (1)
Timing of intervention	Immediately before stimulus (1)
Participants (individual; group)	Group (2)
Medium of intervention (person, videotape, play book, medication)	Person (1) Play (3)
Outcome measure (physiological, behavioral, self-report)	Pulse rate (1); blood pressure (1); behavioral (3)
Type of statistical test used	ANOVA (3)
Critical value	F = 2.53

book should be developed and used in the review of several research reports. Revisions should be made as needed before the actual coding process begins.

CRITICAL EVALUATION OF THE RESEARCH

A critical analysis of studies in an integrative review or meta-analysis requires an organized approach to evaluating the rigor and substance of each study. Some authors recommended excluding certain studies a priori (Eysenck, 1978), whereas others have called for inclusion of all studies (Glass & Smith, 1978; Smith & Naftel, 1984). Smith and Naftel (1984) recommended coding the quality of various dimensions of the study and statistically analyzing whether the quality is related to other variables. For instance, in a meta-analysis the adequacy of the design of a study is reflected in low quality ratings. These ratings can be used to weigh the overall contribution of the study when calculating effect sizes.

In the Broome, Lillis, and Smith (1989) meta-analysis the 73-item Quality of Study Instrument was used, which required the researchers to rate each of 15 categories across four dimensions (see Table 12–5). It is necessary to have more than one individual rate the quality of studies to reduce subjectivity and bias (Stock, Okun, Horning, Miller, Kinney, & Ceuvorst, 1982). Two raters are needed to complete the codebook as well as the quality ratings but are especially important in the quality of study ratings because most instruments available require some degree of interpretation. In fact, Broome, Lillis, and Smith (1989) found they had to develop definitions of several terms in the Quality of Study Instrument they used in order to achieve satisfactory levels of interrater reliability.

Separate estimates of interrater reliability, using accepted statistical procedures, should be computed for both the codebook and the Quality of Study Instrument. Any quality of study tool should evaluate all steps of the research process as reflected in a publication. Essential elements include adequacy of the literature review, design considerations, instrumentation, analysis, and conclusions. Ratings could vary from "present or not" to a five-point Likert-type scale. The less variability in response options, of course, the more restricted the range of quality scores and the less they contribute to any analysis.

The raters using the Quality of Study Instrument should be trained and should practice until they meet a preset standard determined by the investigator (e.g., 90 percent agreement). Subsequent quality scores must be interpreted carefully, as they can be affected by several factors. A quality score is somewhat reflective of the amount of information provided in the study. In published research, space limitations often preclude the inclusion of some information. This is one reason dissertation quality scores are generally higher than published articles. Another factor that influences quality scores is the familiarity of the rater with the area of study. If a rater is familiar with the area, it is easy to read between the lines and unintentionally inflate

Table 12-5   *Quality of Study Instrument*

ELEMENTS AND REQUIREMENTS	1 LOW	2 MED	3 HIGH	0 ABSENT	NA
1.0 *Introduction*					
1.1 Justification for study					
1.2 Conceptual framework					
1.3 Statement of problem or purpose					
1.4 Critical review of issues					
1.5 Methodological issues					
1.6 Hypotheses or study questions stated					
1.7 Operational definitions					
			Sum = _____	n = _____	
2.0 *Methodology*					
2.1 Design described					
2.2 Control of validity threats					
2.3 Sufficient sample size					
2.4 Representative sample					
2.5 Data collection procedures described					
2.6 Instrument validity described					
2.7 Instrument reliability described					
			Sum = _____	n = _____	
3.0 *Data Analysis and Results*					
3.1 Statistical treatment					
3.2 Data presentation					

Continued.

Table 12–5   Quality of Study Instrument   Continued

ELEMENTS AND REQUIREMENTS	1 LOW	2 MED	3 HIGH	0 ABSENT	NA
3.3 Results related to problem and/or hypotheses					
3.4 Findings are substantiated by methods used				Sum = ____	n = ____
4.0 Conclusions/Recommendations					
4.1 Discussion related to background and significance					
4.2 Conclusions logically derived from findings/results					
4.3 Recommendations consistent with findings					
4.4 Alternate explanations advanced					
				Sum = ____	n = ____
				n = ____	
				Sum = ____	
				Mean = ____	

From Smith, M.C., & Stullenbarger, E. (1992). A prototype for integrative review and meta-analysis of nursing research. *Journal of Advanced Nursing, 16*(11), 1272–1283.

a score. A third consideration arises when both published and unpublished information are used. Quality scores, as a whole, may be higher in meta-analyses that include only published material than in those that use all sources, and more importantly, they may lack variability, which will make any analysis related to quality scores less meaningful.

Analysis and Synthesis in Integrative Reviews

The process of conducting integrative reviews and meta-analyses differ somewhat at the point of analysis. Analysis has been defined as "the categorization, ordering, manipulating, and summarizing of data to obtain answers to research questions" (Kerlinger, 1973, p. 134). In most integrative reviews this categorization, ordering, and summarizing of the data is done in a more narrative fashion in which the author attempts to group the major findings of studies by variable of interest. Although there are no standard analysis and interpretation techniques for integrative reviews, most reviewers will present summary conclusions and recommendations for further research based on whether the majority of studies support specific relationships (Cooper, 1989). Meta-analysis, on the other hand, is a method that enables reviews to more closely approximate analytic methods of primary researchers.

Meta-analysis is a relatively new addition to the methods used by scientists to examine the body of knowledge in a specific area (Hedges & Olkin, 1986). Meta-analysis is the application of measurement and statistical techniques to analyze the combined data from multiple studies and the examination of relationships between substantive and methodologic characteristics of the studies and their results (Glass, McGaw, & Smith, 1981). The basic question guiding meta-analyses is "Are there patterns that can be observed in a body of studies in a selected area that have produced a variety of divergent results?" (Bangert-Drowns, 1986).

The term *meta-analysis* was first coined by Glass in 1976. Since that time use of the method has become increasingly widespread, especially in fields such as medicine and nursing, where the effectiveness of interventions must be ascertained, yet subject pools remain small and individual studies are very costly. A large number of studies on a particular intervention provide greater statistical power than any individual study can. In addition, a single study often provides inconclusive findings or even no effect. Yet, other studies of the same phenomenon can yield positive results. It is difficult then to decide which study to use as a guide for practice or for further research (Smith, 1987). Meta-analysis enables a more objective look at the domain of studies and includes as much as possible of the relevant research available.

The conceptual basis for the analysis used in a meta-analysis is based on the transforming of research results from multiple and diverse studies into a common metric representing an index of effect magnitude (Glass, 1976). There are several types of analyses conducted that enable the investigator to describe (1) the scope of the domain, (2) the positive and negative tails of a distribution of studies, (3) any relationships between methodological and substantive variables in the body of studies, and (4) the combined effect of the intervention. Hence, analyses can include descriptive, correlational, analysis of variance, combined probability tests, and effect size estimates.

SCOPE OF THE DOMAIN

Descriptive statistics are usually used to provide a perspective of what literature comprises the area (i.e., year of publication, authors, and disciplines, etc.). These are also used to describe the positive and negative tails of the distribution (i.e., distribution of effect size estimates). Effect size estimates are calculated to examine the strength of the relationship or treatment and its practical importance and meaningfulness (Wolf, 1986). Correlational procedures are used as well as analysis of variance and regression techniques to determine relationships between selected substantive and methodologic variables. Broome, Lillis, and Smith (1989), in their meta-analysis of pediatric pain management interventions, found a difference between the quality of study ratings and the type of publication (dissertation or journal). Nevertheless, ANOVA procedures revealed no significant differences between the type of intervention (books, play, etc.) and children's responses to pain.

DETERMINING EFFECT SIZES

Combined probability techniques and effect size estimates have been described in several authoritative texts (Hedges & Olkin, 1985; Rosenthal, 1984; Wolf, 1986). These procedures allow investigators to make conclusions based on a group of studies as opposed to one, or even several, studies. Statistical approaches and techniques have evolved over time and have become more sophisticated. Basically, each technique involves computing an overall effect size for the dependent variable of interest. In some meta-analyses, several effect sizes are computed. For instance, in the meta-analysis of pediatric pain interventions, three separate effect sizes (one for physiological measures, one for behavioral observation measures, and one for self-report of pain) were computed. Certain types of information are needed to perform the analyses for effect size. Although exactly what information is needed depends on the specific statistical procedure used, there are some commonalities. For instance, if one uses the Fisher combined test (Wolf, 1986) the following equation guides the analysis:

$$\chi^2 = -2 \Sigma \log p$$

The exact probability value for each study is necessary to compute this equation. Calculating the exact probability requires the following information: the number of subjects in the study, the statistical test used, and the actual test statistic. The exact probability value can then be computed using the natural logarithm of the exact probability value and multiplying this number by -2. Then all values are summed. The χ^2 statistic is then calculated, with degrees of freedom equal to 2 times the combined number of tests.

An alternative equation, recommended by Rosenthal (1984) and Wolf (1986), uses exact probability values that are converted to standard normal deviations using a table of z values. Then an effect size is obtained using the following formula:

$$z_c = \frac{\Sigma z}{\sqrt{N}}$$

One effect size is calculated for each study, and all are summed; z_c represents the combined z scores. Another important number to calculate is the Fail Safe N (Rosenthal, 1984). This is defined as the number of studies with null results that have not been published (those finding no significant differences between treatment and control groups) that could potentially counterbalance or nullify the results of published studies. The equation used to calculate the Fail Safe N is:

$$1.645 = \frac{K\overline{Z}}{\sqrt{K + X}}$$

where K is the number of studies and $\overline{Z}$ is the mean Z obtained for K. The number of studies needed to raise the effect size probability above .05 level is represented by X. In the Broome, Lillis, and Smith (1989) meta-analysis, this calculation resulted in 649 unpublished studies that reported no significant differences in order to nullify the results.

Issues in Meta-Analysis

There has been a great deal of controversy in the literature in response to the increasing popularity of meta-analysis. Few authors have questioned the need for a more systematic approach to reviewing and evaluating the literature. However, several issues related to combining results of different studies to reach summative conclusions have been identified. These issues center around (1) variable quality of the studies, (2) lack of representativeness in the research reviewed, and (3) variability of outcome measures and independent variables.

Some authors argue that meta-analysis camouflages badly designed studies (Wachter, 1988). This concern is related to the varying quality of different studies. Many meta-analysts have attempted to control for the variability in quality by rating each study (Smith & Naftel, 1984). Others control for this variability by a priori elimination that can reduce already small sample sizes (Lynn, 1989). Most suggest that the researcher use some method of weighting the studies relative to the strength of the design and the reliability and validity of the research, and factor that weighting into an analysis and discussion of findings.

Another concern is related to the representativeness of all studies used (Lynn, 1989). This concern results from the difficulty many meta-analysts have in locating all studies in the population. Some studies have not been published or were conducted as masters theses. Accessing these is time consuming and costly. Yet, journal articles are more likely than unpublished works to contain significant findings. This can result in a positive bias in a meta-analysis when only published studies are used. As noted previously, it is important to keep documentation regarding which literature was accessed and why certain decisions were made throughout the analysis.

A third issue is the concern that variability and subjectivity in instrumentation contribute to invalid results (Sachs, Berrier, Reitman, Ancona-Berk, & Chalmers, 1987). Although many authors of meta-analyses do not address this, others use more than one coder for each study and report interrater reliability estimates for both codebooks and quality of study ratings (Broome, Lillis, & Smith, 1989). If meta-analysis is to be as rigorous as primary research, then it is essential to measure and report reliability of instrumentation when appropriate.

Other criticisms of meta-analysis include the use of only published reviews and the use of studies with different outcome measures in which more than one outcome measure from each study is used to compute an effect size. The latter practice violates most statistical assumptions related to independence and can inflate effect sizes. If more than one finding is used from each study, this gives those particular studies more weight in the overall combined summative statistical conclusions (Bangert-Drowns, 1986; Lynn, 1989). In studies with more than one outcome, the outcomes cannot be assumed to be independent as they are all taken from the same sample. The meta-analyst must decide whether to use only one outcome per study or to calculate different effect sizes for categories of similar outcomes. Each meta-analyst needs to consider all of these criticisms and plan to control for any threats to the validity of their conclusions.

Integrative reviews and meta-analyses are becoming increasingly common in the nursing literature. Both of these methods use a rigorous, systematic approach that parallels the primary research process in searching, selecting, evaluating, and reporting the literature. Research reviews begins with a problem statement and questions that guide the selection of the literature to be evaluated and extraction of information needed to describe the studies and their findings. Whether to conduct an integrative review or a meta-analysis depends on several factors. The first is the questions one wants to answer. If a reviewer wants to know how effective certain interventions are or the overall strength of the relationship between variables, then a meta-analysis will be necessary. But meta-analysis does take some additional knowledge and skill using certain statistical procedures.

Two different attempts have been made to compare a meta-analysis of studies already reported to a previously published narrative review. In the first, Brown and Hellings (1989) conducted a meta-analysis using ten studies on the topic of maternal-infant attachment. They reported a strong positive effect of early contact between mother and infant on later maternal-child attachment. They compared their findings with a previous qualitative review by Lamb and Hwang (1982) who concluded positive effects of early contact were not well supported by empirical evidence. One limitation of this comparison of a meta-analysis and narrative review is that the meta-analysis did not include the same research reviewed in the qualitative review.

McCain and Lynn (1990) conducted a meta-analysis of 29 studies of patient teaching previously reviewed by Wilson-Barnett and Osborne (1983). Only 15 studies from the earlier narrative review reported sufficient data with which to calculate an effect size. Although there were some incongruities between the two analyses, the overall conclusions of both were similar: Patient teaching is clearly beneficial.

It is clear that meta-analysis is a time-consuming, expensive, and somewhat controversial technique. Nevertheless, many of the necessary approaches used in meta-analysis, such as reporting the statistical test and values used to support conclusions, can only improve the traditional approach to reviewing the literature and reporting research (Curlette & Cannella, 1985).

Summary

Integrative reviews are useful when an individual is beginning to build knowledge about a concept. A meta-analysis will be necessary if a reviewer plans to build a research program around a specific concept. Meta-analysis extends the integrative review process to determine cumulative effects of combined results of the studies. These methods will provide nurse scientists with evidence on which to develop future studies to contribute to nursing science and to plan changes in nursing practice.

REFERENCES

Bangert-Drowns, R. (1986). Review of developments in meta-analytic method. *Psychological Bulletin, 99*(3), 388–399.

Beyer, J., & Byers, M. (1985). Knowledge of pediatric pain: The state of the art. *Children's Health Care, 13,* 150–158.

Beyer, J., DeGood, D, Ashley, L., & Russell, G. (1983). Patterns of post-operative analgesic use with adults and children following cardiac surgery. *Pain, 17,* 71–81.

Broome, M., Lillis, P., & Smith, M. (1989). Pain interventions with children: A meta-analysis. *Nursing Research, 38*(3), 154–158.

Brown, M., & Hellings, P. (1989). A case study of qualitative versus quantitative reviews: The maternal-infant bonding controversy. *Journal of Pediatric Nursing, 4*(2), 104–111.

Burns, N., & Grove, S. (1987). *The practice of nursing research: Conduct, critique and utilization.* Philadelphia: W.B. Saunders.

Burokas, L. (1985). Factors affecting nurses' decisions to medicate pediatric patients after surgery. *Heart and Lung, 14,* 373–379.

Cooper, H. (1987). Literature searching strategies of integrative research reviewers: A first survey. *Knowledge, 8,* 372–383.

Cooper, H. (1989). *Integrating research: A guide for literature reviews.* Beverly Hills: Sage.

Crane, J. (1969). Social structure in a group of scientists: A test of the "invisible college" hypothesis. *American Psychological Review, 34,* 335–352.

Curlette, W., & Cannella, K. (1985). Going beyond the narrative summarization of research findings: The meta-analysis approach. *Research in Nursing and Health, 8,* 293—301.

Eland, J., & Anderson, C. (1977). The experience of pain in children. In A. Jacox (Ed.), Pain: A sourcebook for nurses and other professionals (pp. 453–473). Boston: Little, Brown.

Eysenck, H. (1978). An exercise in siblings. *American Psychologist, 33,* 17.

Fernandez, E., & Turk, D. (1989). The utility of cognitive coping strategies for altering pain perception: A meta-analysis of pain. *Pain, 38*(2), 123–135.

Fullerton, J.T., & Wingard, D. (1990). Methodological problems in the assessment of nurse-midwifery practice. *Applied Nursing Research, 3*(4), 153–160.

Gadish, H. (1988). Factors affecting nurses' decisions to administer pediatric pain medication postoperatively. *Journal of Pediatric Nursing, 3,* 388–390.

Ganong, L. (1987). Integrative reviews of nursing research. *Research in Nursing and Health, 10,* 1–11.

Glass, G.V. (1976). Primary, secondary, and meta-analysis of research. *The Educational Researcher, 5,* 1083–1088.

Glass, G.V., McGaw, B., & Smith, M.L. (1981). *Meta-analysis in social research.* Beverly Hills: Sage.

Glass, G., & Smith, M. (1978). Reply to Eysenek. *American Psychologist, 33,* 517–518.

Hedges L., & Olkin, I. (1985). *Statistical methods for meta-analysis.* Orlando, Fla: Academic Press.

Hedges, L., and Olkin I. (1986). Meta-analysis: A review and new view. *Educational Research, 3,* 14–21.

Kerlinger, F.N. (1973). *Foundations of behavioral research* (2nd ed.). New York: Holt, Rinehart & Winston.

Lamb, M., & Hwang, C. (1982). Maternal-attachment and mother-neonate bonding: A critical review. In M.E. Lamb and A.L. Brown (Eds.), *Advances in developmental psychology* (Vol. 2, pp. 1–39). Hillsdale, NJ: Erlbaum.

Lynn, M. (1989). Meta-analysis: Appropriate tool for the integration of nursing research. *Nursing Research, 38,* 302–305.

Mather, L., & Mackie, J. (1983). The incidence of post-operative pain in children. *Pain, 15,* 271–282.

McCain, N., & Lynn, M. (1990). Meta-analysis of a narrative review: Studies evaluating patient teaching. *Western Journal of Nursing Research, 12,* 347–358.

McCain, N., Smith, M., & Abraham, J. (1986). Meta-analysis of nursing interventions: The codebook as a research instrument. *Western journal of nursing research, 8,* 153–167.

Rosenthal, K. (1984). *Meta-analysis procedures for social science research.* Beverly Hills: Sage.

Sachs, H.S., Berrier, J., Reitman, D., Ancona-Berk, V.A., & Chalmers, T.C. (1987). Meta-analysis of randomized controlled trials. New England Journal of Medicine, *316,* 450–455.

Scholarly Communication: Report of the National Enquiring. (1979). Baltimore: John Hopkins University Press.

Smith, M.C. (1987). Meta-analysis: Conceptual issues. In S. Gortner (Ed.), *Nursing science methods: A reader.* San Francisco: School of Nursing, University of California.

Smith, M.C., & Naftel, D. (1984). Meta-analysis: A perspective for research synthesis. *Image, 16,* 9–13.

Stock, W., Okun, M., Horning, M., Miller, W., Kinney, C., & Ceuvorst, R. (1982). Region in data synthesis: A case of reliability in meta-analysis. *Educational Research, 11*(6), 10–14, 20.

Thompson, R. (1990). Vulnerability in research: A development perspective on research risk. *Child Development, 61,* 1–16.

Tuckman, B. (1978). *Conducting educational research.* New York: Hartcourt, Brace, Jovanovich.

Wachter, K. (1988). Disturbed by meta-analysis. *Science, 241,* 1407–1408.

Wilson, H. (1985). *Research in nursing.* Menlo Park, Calif: Addison-Wesley.

Wilson-Barnett, J., & Osborne *[sic; Oborne],* J. (1983). Studies evaluating patient teaching: Implications for practice. *International Journal of Nursing Studies, 20,* 33–44.

Wolf, F. (1986). Meta-analysis: Quantitative methods for research synthesis. Beverly Hills: Sage.

Woods, N. (1988). Analyzing existing knowledge. In M. Woods and M. Catanzaro (Eds.), *Research: Theory and practice.* St. Louis: Mosby.

Woods, N., Yates, B., & Primomo, J. (1989). Supporting families during chronic illness. *Image, 21,* 46–30.

Chapter 13

Concept Development in Nursing Diagnosis

NANCY S. CREASON, DOROTHY D. CAMILLERI, AND MI JA KIM

*T*he advent of nursing diagnosis is regarded by some as one of the most important developments in nursing over the past two decades (Fitzpatrick, 1989). This recognition is based on political and professional considerations, rather than evaluations of its level of development as theory, or its current conceptual clarity. Nursing diagnosis is a problem-centered approach to planning for the nursing care requirements of particular individuals. When properly developed, it will allow nurses to tie the individual's signs and symptoms to a diagnostic label, and the label to a meaningful course of nursing action. Thus, it is a useful framework for guiding nursing practice and for organizing the knowledge upon which practice is built.

As an approach to guiding nursing practice, the significance of nursing diagnosis lies in its interconnection with goals that have a priority status on the nursing profession's agenda. It provides a vehicle for communicating with various publics about the health problems nurses are prepared to manage, and the specific services nurses can offer in response to the presence of actual or potential health problems. It is regarded by many as a cornerstone in nursing's quest for recognition as independent, autonomous practitioners and in negotiations with third-party payers (private insurers and the government) for reimbursement for nursing services (Bulechek & McCloskey, 1985; Fitzpatrick, 1989; Kim, Camilleri, & Mortensen, 1991).

These political and professional considerations explain the sense of urgency felt by many nurses about hastening the systematic development of nursing diagnosis. While it is very clear that the potential of nursing diagnosis is great, the developmental work is still at an early stage. The theoretical standing of nursing diagnosis is quite limited, and a number of issues have been raised about the set of nursing diagnoses now available, particularly their conceptual clarity, their fit into a taxonomy, and the kind of scholarship that would best advance their theoretical development.

217

At the 1989 Invitational Conference on Research Methods for Validating Nursing Diagnoses, Knafl (1989) and Gordon (1989) discussed issues of concept development and the potential of concept analysis as a method for developing and refining nursing diagnoses. Gordon underscored the importance of concept development as an area of nursing research and scholarship. Among the focus areas she suggested were the level of generality of diagnostic concepts, their distinctiveness, validity, and their concept-concept relations.

In 1990, Avant echoed the need for scholarship in concept development in her discussion of art and science issues related to nursing diagnosis (Avant, 1990). She identified concept formation and concept formalization as major issues, and called for research programs to validate diagnoses.

In this chapter, we further consider the contribution of *concept analysis* to the scientific development of nursing diagnosis. First we present background information about the terminology of the nursing diagnosis field and the issues in the field that must be addressed. Then we explore the efficacy of various approaches to concept analysis in addressing the issues, report on recent research using concept analysis, and make recommendations for future development.

Terminology and Issues Regarding Nursing Diagnosis

Given the recency of nursing diagnosis, it is perhaps not surprising that a major theme underlying many of the identified issues surrounding it is a lack of clarity or specificity as to how nursing diagnosis knowledge should be structured and the meaning of many of its terms. The working definition adopted by the North American Nursing Diagnosis Association (NANDA) in 1991 states that "Nursing Diagnosis is a clinical judgement about individual, family, or community responses to actual and potential health problems/life processes. Nursing diagnoses provide the basis for selection of nursing interventions to achieve outcomes for which the nurse is accountable." Each diagnosis has a definition; hence, each one is a concept. If diagnoses are judged against a continuum from the highly abstract to the highly concrete, there is considerable variation in level of abstractness among them.

Each nursing diagnosis has three components:
1. The *problem statement,* or nursing diagnosis label plus definition
2. The *etiology* or related factors
3. The signs and symptoms, or *defining characteristics*

The second and third components merit further examination. The signs and symptoms, or defining characteristics, can be regarded as clustering together to form the particular health problem or life process represented or captured by the nursing diagnosis. They serve as indicators for the diagnosis. It is the assessment phase of the nursing process that brings these defining characteristics to the nurse's attention for a nursing diagnosis. Some of them are identified from the subjective reports of patients (for example, patients' perceptions of pain), while others may be discerned from objective clinical information available to the nurse (for example, laboratory reports). Because some characteristics are more essential or universal for a diagnosis than others, attempts have been made by some to establish *essential* or *critical* defining characteristics, or *major* and *minor* defining characteristics. Left unsettled at the present time is the issue of which of the possible defining characteristics are critical and must be present for a diagnosis to be made.

The related factors and etiologies are those conditions that bring about a diagnosis and serve as the focal points for nursing interventions. Therefore, related factors and etiology can be regarded as the proximal antecedents to, or causes of, the problem expressed in the nursing diagnosis.

The following example of the nursing diagnosis *hyperthermia* illustrates first the relationship of the three components to one another and second the overlap in meaning between two of them—the defining characteristics and the related factors. This type of overlap in meaning occurs in many of the currently used diagnoses, and is an important issue to be addressed as nursing diagnoses are further refined. *Hyperthermia* is the nursing diagnostic label attached to the problem defined as "the state in which an individual's body temperature is elevated above his or her normal range" (Kim, McFarland, & McLane, 1991, p. 32). Among the eight related factors listed for it are

- Vigorous activity
- Inappropriate clothing
- Dehydration
- Inability to perspire
- Increased metabolic rate

Contrast these items with the following, listed among the five defining characteristics of the diagnosis:

- Increased respiratory rate
- Flushed skin
- Tachycardia
- Increase in body temperature above the normal range

While it could be argued that the defining characteristics listed are easily identified and measured and therefore can be reliable indicators for hyperthermia, the same might be said of one or two of the related factors. Also, characteristics like tachycardia and increased respiratory rate frequently, though not invariably, lead to flushed skin and an increase in body temperature, a relationship that meets the definition for the related factors or etiology category. To summarize the point, the items within a component category and between the second and third component categories vary in the degree of their abstractness or specificity, and the ease with which they

can be operationalized. Also, some of the items listed as defining characteristics seem to be just as "causal" as items in the related factors category.
Because the related factors or etiologies play a central role in determining
nursing interventions, conceptual clarification between the defining characteristics and the related factors of a diagnosis is essential for sound theoretical development.

The diagnosis *hyperthermia* illustrates another closely related theoretical
concern involving the meaning of *essential* defining characteristics. Questions can be raised about the validity of *tachycardia* and *increased respiratory rate* as essential defining characteristics, since they may be present
in a number of conditions in addition to hyperthermia. Even the *flushed
skin* may be present in some other conditions. At issue here is determining
whether there are single defining characteristics that can be exclusively
associated with a special diagnosis, and whether any single characteristics
would have to be present in all instances of the diagnosis. Rather than
regarding a single characteristic as essential, it may be wiser to regard the
co-occurrence of a set of characteristics as being exclusively associated with
the diagnosis. It may well be useful to combine two ideas: that of a set of
characteristics that are exclusively associated with a diagnosis, and that of
requiring some proportion of items in the set to be present before assigning
the diagnosis. The subgroup of items so selected would have to meet the
criterion of exclusive association—that is, a subgroup would have to indicate only one nursing diagnosis. This plan has two advantages. First, it
would eliminate a possible barrier to the inclusion of highly significant
characteristics that do not occur with great frequency. Second, it would
provide a systematic method for assigning the diagnosis in instances where
all the possible characteristics were not present.

Development of a Taxonomy

The lack of clarity and precision about the meaning of terms that are components for each problem statement or nursing diagnosis also influences a
second commonly identified topic of concern—that of an appropriate taxonomy for nursing diagnosis. Foremost among the issues raised about a
taxonomy for nursing diagnosis are the levels of abstraction either currently
represented or desired, the need for both conceptual and operational definitions, and the conceptual frameworks that should be reflected in the
taxonomy. All these issues touch on concept development or definition,
and it can be said that efforts to develop a taxonomy of nursing diagnoses
are, in effect, efforts toward conceptual definition of nursing diagnosis.

Taxonomy work under the auspices of the North American Nursing Diagnosis Association (NANDA) has been underway since its beginning efforts
at developing nursing diagnosis. The first taxonomic structure was alpha-

betic rather than theoretical. Nurses engaged in this early work focused on specific human functional systems, such as the gastrointestinal system (Gebbie, 1978), and generated diagnoses from their experience and reasoning. Their output, however, was arranged alphabetically rather than by system, and reflected an everyday concept as opposed to scientific concept orientation. This characterization is based on Batey's (1977) and Denzin's (1970) distinction between scientific concepts and everyday concepts. Both help the user to structure his or her environment. However, scientific concepts are "consensually defined within the community of scientists" (Denzin, 1970, p. 39), whereas everyday concepts spring from individual experience and may contain the private unvalidated meanings of the user.

An effective taxonomy for nursing diagnosis would fulfill several conditions. It would contain the broad concepts of a general and abstract nature that would serve as an organizing framework, reflecting the nature of nursing knowledge and providing direction for further knowledge development. Within these broad categories would be concepts of increasingly smaller scope and specificity, representing a logical ordering of concepts from the most general and encompassing to the most specific and narrow in scope. Definitions for these concepts would also be ordered, from the more abstract and general to the more precise and operationalized. Both kinds of definition are needed for the proper development of a nursing diagnosis classification scheme. General or abstract definitions are needed to convey the ideas for which the word label stands. Operational definitions are needed to convey the measurement processes that are followed to recognize the presence of the concept.

Nursing diagnoses would be dispersed throughout the large categories in the taxonomy, and each diagnosis would have some components that were well operationalized, such as the defining characteristics, as well as others that could be less operational. The etiologies, for instance, require careful empirical specification, but this may not entail the same degree of operationalization as would be required for defining characteristics.

At the present time, nursing diagnoses are not well ordered in terms of their level of generality; some diagnoses are very global (anxiety, social isolation) while others are extremely specific (impaired swallowing). The problem is further complicated by the fact that there are overlapping relationships among the component parts of some diagnoses. For example, *decreased cardiac output* is a nursing diagnosis; it may also lead to *activity intolerance,* another nursing diagnosis, which itself is listed as a related factor for still another diagnosis, *mobility, impaired physical.* It is noteworthy that *decreased cardiac output* is most often used in critical care units, while *activity intolerance* and *mobility, impaired physical,* are most often used in ambulatory or community settings. The point is not that overlap of this type is a fatal flaw but that such overlap indicates linked causal chains of events that demand careful consideration in a classification plan. For instance, there may need to be some modification of the commonly held assertion that the nursing intervention for a diagnosis depends to a great extent on the related factors leading to the diagnosis, if indeed a related factor can also *be* a diagnosis.

Two distinct approaches to taxonomy development for nursing diagnosis have been described. Jones (1978) identified five actions as necessary for the task: defining nursing, identifying the data base for each diagnosis, selecting appropriate terminology to label problems (the diagnostic statement), defining the diagnostic terms, and developing a classification system (p. 140). Roy (1980) contended that taxonomies can be developed inductively or deductively and proposed that theory be used to provide an organizing framework for nursing diagnoses (pp. 235–243). The two approaches have gradually merged over the years, as taxonomic work has moved from various levels of abstraction to a more organized, albeit incomplete, hierarchial listing. In 1986, the NANDA Taxonomy Committee (NANDA, 1987) presented Taxonomy I with nine human responses to the membership to be "tested, refined, revised, and expanded" (p. 469). More recently, this taxonomy was revised and coded according to the International Classification of Diseases format (Fitzpatrick et al., 1989).

Some work has also focused on taxonomic validation, a term referring to the establishment of a particular concept as truly representing the consensus of the nursing community about its fit into nursing practice, or as representing a true empirical fit with the clinical manifestations of patients. The work of Coler and colleagues (1989) is an example of validation on a very general level. This work concerned examining the nine human response patterns that were the first level concepts in the NANDA taxonomy, with the goal of determining their utility for psychiatric nursing practice. The group suggested some revisions that they regarded as expanding the usefulness of the taxonomy for their specialty.

The greater proportion of work on the taxonomy reported over the years has concerned the elaboration of the individual nursing diagnoses. Attention has been given to the adequacy of the conceptualization of the patients' problems and the life processes represented, the nature of the related factors and etiologies, and the accuracy of the defining characteristics. The degree of operationalization of all these components has also been a focus. Given this set of issues, it is logical that formalized concept analysis stands out as the method of choice for the further development of nursing diagnosis. Such analysis would help in producing clear conceptual definitions at an appropriate level of empirical specificity. It would also aid in synthesizing information about the use of the concept from all relevant sources, disclosing the degree of consensus already established and pointing to salient areas for future development.

Concept Analysis

Since the early 1980s, concept analysis has been formally presented as an important step in the development of nursing theory (Chinn & Jacobs, 1983; Walker & Avant, 1983). Its importance stems from the position of concepts as the most basic units or building blocks of theory. To the extent that the concepts of a discipline have deficiencies of either faulty or insufficient development, theory building for the discipline will be less robust than would be desirable. This necessary focus on concepts as the foundation of theory development has called attention to various means of establishing and explicating the meaning of concepts. Concept analysis is one means of doing so, and has been described at the most generic level by Knafl and Deatrick, in chapter 3, as synthesizing existing views of a concept, and distinguishing the concept from all others.

Concept analysis rests on several assumptions about the nature of concepts that bear examination. First, concepts are a human creation. That is, the *meaning* dimension of a concept is not an inherent property of it, simply waiting to be discovered. The meaning is instead an invention of its users. A concept is invested with whatever meaning serves the purposes of its users.

Second, concepts consist of interrelated components. Included are the word label or symbol, the ideas or cognitions represented by the label, and some empirical events, referents, or phenomena connected to the idea and the label. A concept is not synonymous with a human experience; it can convey a mental image of a human experience, however, or have human experience as an indicator or a reference point. Concepts are also quite distinct from phenomena. In fact, Gordon (1989) points out that a clinical phenomenon can look very different when different theoretical or conceptual perspectives are applied. As an example, the same patient behavior may be regarded as "decisional conflict" by one person, and indifference or even "powerlessness" by another. The concepts applied to a phenomenon influence what the user discerns about the phenomenon. Third, concepts are so constructed that it is possible to tell which ideas and empirical phenomena are included in them, as well as which are excluded.

Nursing concepts are those that capture or represent phenomena in the domain of nursing. For example, one might identify *health* and *caring* as nursing concepts. Nursing diagnosis concepts are a specific subclassification of nursing concepts. They are intended to serve the purpose of representing a patient's problem or life process in a way that can be tied to a set of nursing interventions designed to ameliorate or manage the problem. They also provide a common language for communicating about patients, thus facilitating consistency in nursing care. These purposes will influence some of the choices that can be made in how the concepts can best be developed.

Models of Concept Analysis

Several models of concept analysis have been described, including those by Chinn and Jacobs (now Kramer) (1983, 1991), Walker and Avant (1983, 1988), Sartori (1984), Rodgers (1989), and Schwartz Barcott and Kim (1986). At an early point in the analytical process, all these models call for a review of the literature on the concept being analyzed. A literature review is also the most common element of analysis to be found in work on nursing diagnosis, whether or not the scholars regard themselves as conducting a concept analysis. Because of the ultimate use of the concept for describing patient problems that are amenable to nursing intervention, a distinction is frequently made between the usage found in the nursing literature and usage found in other related literature. Caution must be exercised in incorporating nonnursing sources, since some concepts may be used differently by various disciplines. These sources are most useful in calling to nurse scholars' attention the full range of meaning associated with the use of a concept, and they can be invaluable sources of enrichment in deciding upon the meanings most useful for incorporation into the nursing meaning.

CHINN AND JACOBS

Models of concept analysis differ in their portrayal of the emphases and function of the literature review. Chinn and Jacobs (Kramer) (1983, 1991), for instance, call for at least a tentative identification of the concept of interest to begin the analysis. They state as the purpose of analysis, to "produce a tentative definition of the concept and a set of tentative criteria for determining if the concept 'exists' in a particular situation" (1983, p. 80). Rather than emphasizing details about how the literature review should be done, they stress the need for the analyst to acquire from various sources the array of meanings or definitions currently in use for the concept. These meanings yield the criteria that are used for the concept in one of two ways. They are needed for recognizing the concept's presence, in those instances where the analysis begins with an actual model case. These meanings are also needed for the more typical procedure, the construction of cases for the concept. Several cases are constructed and refined as the analysis proceeds, including the model case, a contrary case, and a borderline or related case. A testing phase follows, consisting of a flexible but very logical examination of similarities and differences among the cases, with emphasis on practical, empirical considerations. This testing process leads to refinement of both the general meaning and specific criteria that are desirable to include for the model case. Ultimately, all necessary and sufficient criteria are identified from iterations of the process.

The Chinn and Jacobs (Kramer) model was followed in the analyses conducted by Forsyth (1980) on empathy, and by Knafl and Deatrick (1986) on normalization, neither of which are nursing diagnoses. Forsyth noted that rather than being exhaustive, her literature review was targeted toward authors (or other usages) that facilitate the extraction of meaning about the concept. She noted that literature from a broad range of fields of inquiry is sought to test the consistency—or lack thereof—of conceptualizations in various fields. Both analyses had as a purpose to distinguish their concept from others that were sometimes confused with it.

The cases that the Chinn and Jacobs (Kramer) guidelines call for can be either from clinical experience or constructed to utilize all relevant criteria. Because of the nature of nursing diagnosis concepts, most experts would argue that the cases used in at least advanced stages of the analysis come from clinical settings, and that the criteria be empirical and lend themselves to operationalization.

WALKER AND AVANT

The guidelines of Walker and Avant (1983, 1988) for concept analysis also start with the selection of a concept of interest, and proceed to determining the specific aims or purposes of the analysis. The aims of the analysis are critical, since at a later point in the analysis, they will become the basis upon which decisions are made about the selection of appropriate defining characteristics or attributes. The review of the literature and other sources for information about current meanings and usages of the concept is set forth as exhaustive rather than targeted. Once the plethora of possible meanings, definitions, and characteristics are examined, the investigator sifts through them with the particular aims of the analysis in mind, making decisions about which of them should be retained in the final product, based on their contribution to the aims of the project.

Walker and Avant (1988) also call for case construction at the point where the defining attributes seem to be taking shape. Included are model cases, contrary cases, and borderline and related cases. They also describe illegitimate cases (ones where most of the defining attributes will not apply), and invented cases (fanciful nonempirical cases that do, however, illustrate the attributes) as sometimes used. Analysis and comparison across all of these cases helps with the refinement of the concept and its defining characteristics. The process is expected to eliminate vagueness, overlap among attributes, or contradiction between attributes and the model case.

Two further steps are included in Walker and Avant's (1988) guidelines, both of which seem valuable for analysis of nursing diagnosis concepts. They are first, the identification of the antecedents and the consequences of the concept, and second, the determination of the empirical referents for the critical attributes. Identifying the antecedents and consequences of a nursing diagnosis concept has been an outstanding need in the field of nursing diagnosis, expressed as the need to link etiologies to the signs and symptoms or defining characteristics of these diagnoses, and further, to the nursing interventions specific to the etiologies. The need for well-defined empirical referents for linking these aspects of nursing diagnosis into a unified package has also been firmly established.

According to Walker and Avant (1988), the literature review for a concept is very broad based. Therefore, Walker and Avant's guidelines provide a good format for accessing and taking advantage of other disciplines' views or compilation of information about a concept, while maintaining a strong focus on the utility of the information for dealing with phenomena that nurses encounter.

Although the analysis of the concept *intuition* by Rew (1986) follows Walker and Avant's guidelines and does consider antecedents, consequences, and limited empirical referents for the concept, the resulting definition of the concept remains on a somewhat general level, and was not elaborated in such a way as to yield the defining characteristics and related factors or etiologies associated with a nursing diagnosis.

SARTORI

Sartori's (1984) method for concept analysis emphasizes the refinement, or "reconstruction" of concepts, using a three-stage approach (reconstruction, naming, and reconceptualization) and relying on literature sources for data, rather than constructing cases or identifying actual empirical cases to exemplify the concept. Because Sartori's method does not involve any form of empirical validation for the newly synthesized concept, it has less utility for developing nursing diagnoses than other models of concept analysis. The method does provide a sound and systematic means for examining the various uses of a concept to be found in the literature, and therefore may be helpful in arriving at the initial specification of theoretical underpinnings, etiologies, or defining characteristics for the nursing diagnosis concept. An investigator would need to add some empirical steps for validating the concept so developed.

RODGERS

Rodgers' (1989) recommendations for concept analysis have some similarities and differences compared to the methods already described. The fundamental purpose of concept analysis, for Rodgers, is to clarify the current status of a concept of interest. The analysis does so by examining the historical or evolutionary background of the concept and by determining areas of agreement and disagreement among various disciplines in the use of the concept. A distinctive feature of her view is the portrayal of the meaning of concepts as changing or evolving over time. She also describes the analytical process as a series of overlapping phases rather than a set of sequential steps. Her view is similar to that of Walker and Avant (1983) in explicitly attending to the antecedents and consequences of the concept as part of the analytical process. The analysis deals with both the extant meanings of the concept, as well as an assessment of changes that have taken place over time. Because of the evolutionary and interrelated nature of concepts, Rodgers advocates developing only a model case, rather than borderline or contrary cases. The use of the latter two categories she regards as investing the concept with a degree of stability or unchangability and isolation that it does not possess. She prefers to discuss *related concepts,* since that term implies the interconnectedness of the world and the likelihood of change and allows the analyst to discriminate between those attributes illustrating the model case and those that are, instead, indicators of a different (though close) concept. For instance, in an analysis of grief, Cowles and Rodgers (1991) identify *bereavement* and *mourning* as related concepts. Rodgers also advocates identifying actual cases, rather than artificially constructing them.

The Cowles and Rodgers (1991) analysis of the concept of grief was undertaken with its status and future potential as a nursing diagnosis in mind. As evidenced in this work, Rodgers' guidelines are quite explicit about the methods to be followed to enhance the scientific credibility of the final product. For instance, it is stated that a literature sample of about 20 percent of the total population, or at least 30 items, is sufficient to identify convergence in the data (p. 120). Detailed descriptions of literature sampling and inductive analytical procedures are also offered.

In the analysis of grief, several attributes of grief were discerned from the sample of literature chosen for the study, leading to the depiction of grief as "a *dynamic, pervasive,* highly *individualized process* with a strong *normative* component (the italicized words are the attributes). Both antecedents and consequences of grief were identified from the sample of literature chosen. The discussion of the evolution of grief was based on a purposive sample of six classic works that had been cited most often in the literature included in the regular sample. In their discussion, the authors point to the difficulty of identifying a grief response in reference to a finite set of defining characteristics, because of its highly individualized and pervasive nature. They identify the need for further research based on in-depth interviews as a primary data source, to arrive at a specific conceptualization of grief as it is experienced by people receiving nursing care. Without such understanding, attempts to identify unique cases of grief such as *dysfunctional* or *anticipatory* are premature.

Much of the work published in the nursing diagnosis literature has followed certain aspects of the concept analysis guidelines described above, with varying degrees of attention to an empirical phase, either for initial development, or for validation. More specifically, nurse investigators have used the literature and the expert opinions of practitioners (informally or through surveys) to gather information about the nursing diagnosis concept. In some instances, a broad range of information was gathered, including theoretical definitions, information about the range of etiologies and signs and symptoms, and whatever operational definitions were possible. In other instances, a more restricted review of the literature was undertaken. Investigators may or may not have had, as part of their methodology, an empirical phase. When present, the empirical phase has involved surveys of nurses for their clinical judgments about the defining characteristics of a diagnosis, or nurse assessments of a clinical patient population to validate that the patients *do,* indeed, demonstrate the defining characteristics.

EXAMPLES IN NURSING DIAGNOSIS LITERATURE

Two examples of nursing diagnoses analyses are presented here to illustrate the range in emphases to be found. The diagnoses are anxiety and alterations in urinary elimination. The two analyses represent different investigative approaches. The first is an article by Whitley (1989) on anxiety, an important nursing diagnosis that can be characterized as diffuse and lacking in clarity because of interrelated factors such as its abstractness, lack of clear empirical referents, and lack of operational definitions. It is therefore difficult to distinguish between it and other closely related concepts such as fear. Whitley's work emphasized the validation of defining characteristics for this diagnosis. From the literature she presented four theoretical definitions of anxiety from nonnursing sources: psychoanalytic, behavioral, interpersonal, and biologic. Whitley then refers to the Peplau (1986) work on anxiety presented in the book *Some Clinical Approaches to Psychiatric Nursing* (Burd & Marshall, 1986); definitions of anxiety commonly found in nursing also were reviewed. Whitley then summarized and discussed the findings of several validation studies for the concept. The point of these validation studies was to secure a reasonable level of consensus about the defining characteristics for the nursing diagnosis, anxiety.

Included among the studies Whitley reviewed were four surveys of nurses to elicit their judgments about which of the following characteristics were sufficiently common to be retained as defining characteristics. Also included were three studies (Aukamp, 1986; Fadden, Fehring, & Rossi, 1987; Kim et al., 1984) in which nurse clinicians assessed a sample of patients to identify the presence of defining characteristics. Cardiovascular patients, unspecified medical surgical patients, and third trimester antepartum patients comprised the samples for these studies. The antepartum patient study included responses from the study patients themselves ($N = 30$) and included contributing factors as well as defining characteristics. Four of the studies utilized the Fehring standard of requiring a 75 percent (later changed to 80 percent) or above agreement among raters about the presence of a defining characteristic before it could be considered a critical defining characteristic, or indicator, of the diagnosis. In all four, the characteristics *anxious* and *apprehension* met that requirement. In addition, *increased tension* and *worried* met the requirement in three of the four studies. In her discussion, Whitley points out the need for the comparison of findings across a number of studies, as well as for further empirical validation studies for the concept, using clinical specialists instead of less expert registered nurses.

The findings Whitley reported could also support an argument for more concerted concept analysis before proceeding with the validation phase. The presence of *anxious* as a defining characteristic of anxiety was strikingly circular and suggested that the concept was insufficiently refined for maximum utility as a nursing diagnosis. Although four theoretical perspectives were given about the sources or causes of anxiety, little attention was paid to the parameters of anxiety as a clinical phenomenon, its empirical manifestations and related factors, and measurement issues and operational definitions for these manifestations. The validation studies presented are most useful for establishing whether a characteristic is seen with sufficient frequency to be included as a defining characteristic, and may therefore eliminate some possible choices (*regretful* is one such characteristic that was eliminated for the nursing diagnosis anxiety). A sound analysis with particular emphasis on empirical referents of various aspects of the concept, and on operational definitions where possible, may well improve the clinical significance of the characteristics and related factors that are to be validated.

Voith's (1986) work on alterations in urinary elimination reflects a different analytical perspective. She concentrates on analyzing the concept of altered urinary elimination, with an emphasis on understanding the underlying anatomical or physiological dysfunctions, some empirical indicators of that dysfunction, the signs and symptoms, and some possible etiologies. This comprehensive assessment relies heavily on targeted literature from nonnursing sources, and does not include an empirical phase for validating any defining characteristics or etiologies and related factors that are evidence for the diagnosis. She uses the analysis, instead, to collate and assess information already in the literature, and to demonstrate that alterations in urinary elimination should have the status of a diagnostic category that contains the more precisely defined subcategories of urinary retention, on the one hand, and urinary incontinence on the other. Urinary incontinence would be further categorized into stress incontinence, urge incontinence, reflex incontinence, and uncontrolled incontinence. These breakdowns reflect the differing etiologies, which in turn, require differing nursing interventions.

Both of the above examples illustrate sound investigative work though the emphases (or aims) and nature of the product are different. Both products are needed for development of nursing diagnoses, and ideally, investigations into nursing diagnoses would combine these approaches. The need to combine various empirical approaches with analytical approaches to concept development has led to a burgeoning of interest in another recently defined model for concept analysis developed by Schwartz-Barcott and Kim (1986).

THE HYBRID MODEL OF CONCEPT ANALYSIS

Schwartz-Barcott and Kim (1986) have named their model for concept analysis the *hybrid model* because it combines the essential elements of two contrasting approaches to concept development, both of which are needed for adequate specification and elaboration of concepts dealing with nursing phenomena. It is specifically designed to draw on insights from clinical practice. The model combines a theoretical approach, in which various extant meanings or uses of a concept are examined, evaluated, and synthesized, with an empirical approach, focusing on actual observations of clinical phenomena as inductive data sources for generating and developing concepts.

The model has three phases beginning with the theoretical, progressing to a fieldwork phase, and culminating in a final analytical phase. As with other models for concept analysis, there is considerable movement and overlap of phases.

In the theoretical phase, the concept is selected, the literature reviewed, and finally, a working definition tentatively agreed upon. Selecting the concept is characterized by breadth and flexibility; new concepts may be generated from encounters with patients in a nursing practice situation, or already known concepts may be drawn directly from other disciplines or the nursing literature. The source is unimportant, if the concept is relevant to a phenomenon of interest to nursing. Consistent with this emphasis, a hybrid model literature search is broad rather then narrow and is focused on providing answers to questions about definition and measurement. The aim is to gather as much information as possible about currently held meanings for the concept. As part of the analysis occurring in this phase, the authors recommend that attention be paid to the status of a concept as either an independent, or a dependent variable. This recommendation is very much in keeping with the need in nursing diagnosis for establishing causal linkages and for reflecting these linkages in the taxonomy.

The hybrid model fieldwork phase is designed to bring the investigator into clinical encounters with patients or settings that exemplify the concept under development. This phase draws on the traditional inductive approaches to theory generation and the research techniques common to natural field studies, such as participant observation. Attention is paid to selecting a setting and cases that provide opportunity for frequent observations of the phenomena of interest. Emphasis is placed on having a very limited, rather than large, number of carefully chosen cases, that are studied in depth. During this phase, a model case, a contrary case, and a borderline case are chosen. These cases are useful in clarifying and refining aspects of the concept, and in discovering good empirical indicators and, sometimes, measurement techniques for the concept. The hybrid model culminates in a final analysis phase, in which there is an integration of the findings of the fieldwork phase with the earlier theoretical phase.

The attention given in a hybrid model to actual empirical cases as they occur in clinical settings can be helpful in achieving the operational definitions so needed for the development of sound nursing diagnoses. Gordon (1989) suggested that this model with its qualitative field methods can be useful in conducting taxonomic analysis for those nursing diagnoses that are so broad, they are higher taxonomic categories rather than nursing diagoses. She offered *altered skin integrity* and *parental role conflict* as examples of diagnoses in need of such analysis.

Of central importance in the hybrid model as developed by Schwartz-Barcott and Kim is the emphasis on the qualitative nature of the fieldwork phase. Other nursing diagnosis investigators have developed methodologies for validation studies in nursing diagnoses that share some of the principles enunciated by Schwartz-Barcott and Kim, but differ with regard to the reliance on qualitative research methods for the fieldwork phase of the analysis.

Lo and Kim (1986) report on their methodological study to develop construct validity of the nursing diagnosis sleep pattern disturbance, in the Proceedings of the Sixth NANDA conference. They regard their work as a modified version of Schwartz-Barcott and Kim's (1986) hybrid model because of the striking similarities in methodology between the two, even though they were developed independently over a roughly similar time period. The major difference between the hybrid model and the modification followed by Lo and Kim lies in the aims and procedures used in the fieldwork or clinical investigation phase. Lo and Kim's study began with an extensive literature review on sleep pattern disturbance that provided both the theoretical underpinning and an exhaustive list of 33 defining characteristics for the concept. They then proceeded to a two-stage clinical investigation phase to validate the clinical relevance of these defining characteristics for the nursing diagnosis sleep pattern disturbance. The first stage used expert nurse ratings to validate the proposed defining characteristics, and the second stage involved clinical assessments of patients, to detect the presence or absence of the defining characteristics.

The final analysis section of Lo and Kim's work with sleep pattern disturbance also reflected some differences in method, if not in aims, from the Schwartz-Barcott and Kim model. Lo and Kim's final analysis subjected the data from the earlier phase to statistical techniques to check for homogeneity among the defining characteristics, and for their patterns of occurrence in the patient group. Based on this analysis, some items were retained, while others were discarded because they did not occur with sufficient frequency to warrant retention as defining characteristics.

Summary

Because of its clinical and professional relevance, nursing diagnosis is becoming one of the more important areas of emphasis for nurse scholars, and concept analysis is recommended as an effective means for addressing some of the developmental issues encountered in its scientific elaboration. The guidelines developed by various authors are useful in arriving at carefully constructed, comprehensive concepts. Since nursing diagnosis is closely tied to nursing interventions designed to eliminate or manage the real or potential problems and life processes experienced by a patient, recommendations about particular aspects of the analysis to be emphasized can be made. Perhaps most important is the need for inclusion of explicit validation phases. Some of these would deal with confirming the presence of the proposed defining characteristics of a given nursing diagnosis in patient populations. Others would demonstrate the degree of consensus existing among nurse specialists about the presence, or significance, of the defining characteristics, or of the diagnosis itself. Such emphasis on validation as an integral part of concept analysis would set the stage for the next step on the challenging research agenda for nursing diagnosis—that of connecting specific nursing interventions with the etiologies or related factors leading to the diagnosis, or with the defining characteristics that indicate the diagnosis.

REFERENCES

Aukamp, V. (1986). *Knowledge deficit and anxiety as nursing diagnoses in the third trimester of pregnancy: An exploratory study to identify the defining characteristics and contributing factors.* Unpublished Doctoral Dissertation, University of Texas, Austin.

Avant, K. C. (1990). The art and science in nursing diagnoses development. *Nursing Diagnosis, 1,* 51—56.

Batey, M. V. (1977). Conceptualization: Knowledge and logic guiding empirical research. *Nursing Research, 26,* 324–329.

Bulechek, G. M., McCloskey, J. C. (1985). Future directions. In G. M. Bulechek & J. C. McCloskey (Eds.), *Nursing interventions: Treatments for nursing diagnoses* (pp. 401–408). Philadelphia: WB Saunders.

Chinn, P. L., & Jacobs, M. K. (1983). *Theory and nursing: A systematic approach.* St. Louis: Mosby.

Chinn, P. L., & Kramer, M. K. (1991). *Theory and nursing: A systematic approach* (3rd ed.). St. Louis: Mosby.

Coler, M. S., Johnson, T., Amaro, A., Johnson, B., Snayd, J., Wiedliyer, C., Caplan, C., Dodge, J., Lee, J., & Thayer, K. (1989). NANDA Taxonomy I: A preliminary validation/invalidation study. In R. M. Carroll-Johnson (Ed.), *Classification of nursing diagnoses: Proceedings of the eighth conference* (pp. 141–151). Philadelphia: Lippincott.

Cowles, K. V., & Rodgers, B. L. (1991). The concept of grief: A foundation of nursing research and practice. *Research in Nursing & Health, 14,* 119–127.

Denzin, J. K. (1970). *The research act: A theoretical introduction to sociological methods.* Chicago: Aldine.

Fadden, T., Fehring, R., & Rossi, E. (1987). Clinical validation of the diagnosis anxiety. In A. M. McLane (Ed.), *Classification of nursing diagnoses: Proceedings of the seventh conference.* St. Louis: Mosby.

Fitzpatrick, J. J. (1989). Conceptual basis for the organization and advancement of nursing knowledge: Nursing diagnosis/taxonomy. *Proceedings for the 1989 National Forum on Doctoral Education in Nursing* (pp. 33–34). Indianapolis: Indiana University School of Nursing.

Fitzpatrick, J. J., Kerr, M., Saba, V. K., Hoskins, L., Hurley, M., Mills, W., Rottkamp, B., & Warren, J. J. (1989). NANDA Taxonomy I: Proposed ICD-CD 10 Version. *Applied Nursing Research, 2,* 90–91.

Forsyth, G. L. (1980). Analysis of the concept of empathy: Illustration of one approach. *Advances in Nursing Science, 2*(2), 33–42.

Gebbie, K. M. (1978). Toward the theory development for nursing diagnosis classification. In M. J. Kim & D. A. Mortiz (Eds.), *Classification of nursing diagnosis: Proceedings of the third and fourth national conferences* (pp. 8–12). New York: McGraw-Hill.

Gordon, M. (1989). Response to K. Knafl's paper on concept development. *Monograph of the invitational conference on research methods for validating nursing diagnoses.* St. Louis: NANDA.

Jones, P. E. (1978). Determining terminology: A University of Toronto experience. In M. J. Kim & D. A. Moritz (Eds.), *Classification of nursing diagnoses: Proceedings of the third and fourth national conferences* (pp. 138–145). New York: McGraw-Hill.

Kim, M. J., Camilleri, D. D., & Mortensen, R. A. (1991). Nursing diagnosis and nursing practice: Dialogue with Nordic nurses. *Nursing Science & Research in the Nordic Countries, 21*(11), 30–33.

Kim, M. J., McFarland, G. K., & McLane, A. M. (1991). *Pocket guide to nursing diagnoses* (4th ed.). St. Louis: Mosby.

Kim, M. J., Seritella, R. A., Gulanick, M., Moyer, K., Parsons, E., Scherbel, J., Stafford, M., Suhayda, R., & Yocum, C. (1984). Clinical validation of cardiovascular nursing diagnoses. In M. J. Kim, G. K. McFarland, A. M. McLane (Eds.), *Classification of nursing diagnoses: Proceedings of the fifth national conference.* St. Louis: Mosby.

Knafl, K. (1989). Concept Development. *Monograph of the Invitational Conference on Research Methods for Validating Nursing Diagnoses.* St. Louis: NANDA.

Knafl, K., & Deatrick, J. (1986). How families manage chronic conditions: An analysis of the concept of normalization. *Research in Nursing and Health, 9,* 215–222.

Lo, C. H., & Kim, M. J. (1986). Construct validity of sleep pattern disturbance: A methodological approach. *Classification of nursing diagnosis: Proceedings of the sixth conference* (pp. 197–206). St Louis: Mosby.

NANDA Taxonomy I. (1987). Guidelines and observations about NANDA nursing diagnosis Taxonomy I. In A. M. McClane (Ed.), *Classification of nursing diagnosis: Proceedings of the seventh conference.* St. Louis: Mosby.

Peplau, H. (1986). A working definition of anxiety. In S. Burd & M. Marshall (Eds.), *Some clinical approaches to psychiatric nursing.* New York: Macmillan.

Rew, L. (1986). Intuition: Concept analysis of a group phenomenon. *Advances in Nursing Science, 8*(2), 21–28.

Rodgers, B. L. (1989). Concepts, analysis and the development of nursing knowledge: The evolutionary cycle. *Journal of Advanced Nursing, 14,* 330–335.

Roy, S. C. (1980). Historical perspective of the theoretical framework of the classification of nursing diagnosis. *Classification of nursing diagnosis: Proceedings of the third and fourth national conferences* (pp. 8–12). New York: McGraw-Hill.

Sartori, G. (1984). Guidelines for concept analysis. In G. Sartori (Ed.), *Social science concepts: A systematic analysis* (pp. 15–85). Beverly Hills: Sage.

Schwartz-Barcott, D., & Kim, H. S. (1986). A hybrid model for concept development. In P. L. Chinn (Ed.), *Nursing research methodology, issues and instrumentation* (pp. 91–101). Rockville, MD: Aspen.

Voith, A. M. (1986, Jan./Feb.). A conceptual framework for nursing diagnoses: Alteration in urinary incontinence. *Rehabilitation Nursing,* 18–21.

Walker, L. O., & Avant, K. C. (1983). *Strategies for theory construction in nursing.* Norwalk, Conn: Appleton-Century-Crofts.

Walker, L. O., & Avant, K. C. (1988). *Strategies for theory construction in nursing* (2nd ed.). Norwalk, Conn: Appleton & Lange.

Whitley, G. G. (1986). *Validation of the nursing diagnosis anxiety: A nurse consensus survey.* Unpublished Doctoral Dissertation, Northern Illinois, University, Dekalb.

Whitley, G. G. (1989). An analysis of the nursing diagnosis anxiety. In R. M. Carroll-Johnson (Ed.), *Classification of nursing diagnosis: Proceedings of the eighth conference* (pp. 371–375). Philadelphia: JB Lippincott.

Chapter 14

Applications and Future Directions for Concept Development in Nursing

BETH L. RODGERS AND KATHLEEN A. KNAFL

A variety of approaches to concept development have been presented in this text. A discussion of the philosophical foundations of concept development provided an overview of some of the major advances associated with this topic over the years. Issues also were identified to assist researchers in selecting techniques appropriate for the intended inquiry and the concept of interest. A comparison of diverse approaches to concept development followed, further enhancing decision making associated with this process.

The methods presented included several distinct approaches to concept analysis, probably the more familiar of the concept development techniques, including Norris's seminal work, along with the simultaneous concept analysis process utilized by Haase and her colleagues to address a domain of related concepts. The hybrid model of Schwartz-Barcott and Kim starts with a systematic literature review and concept analysis and then adds a phase of field research to expand and further clarify the concept through the collection of empirical data in a natural nursing setting. Another approach presented addressed integrated literature reviews, including meta-analysis as a means to develop concepts, probably a less frequently thought of approach that, nonetheless, offers a significant contribution to concept development.

Each of these approaches possesses its own philosophical base, and is oriented toward a specific purpose or outcome. Overall, concept development can be conducted along many lines and in various creative ways. It is fair to say, as well, that it is a never-ending process. A concept may never be completely "finished," but development must continue as new knowledge and experiences emerge. Without continuing effort to develop concepts, progress in nursing may be impeded by a growing quagmire of conceptual problems.

As noted in the introduction to this text, concept development techniques may be just what are needed to resolve significant problems in nursing. However, there is a need to continue evaluating available methods and to create new and innovative approaches to concept development as new problems are identified. The works of Schwartz-Barcott and Kim and Haase and colleagues presented in this book, are excellent examples of recent innovations in concept development techniques. Additional work is needed in several areas, including continued exploration of the nature of concepts, which will shed additional light on appropriate means of development. Similarly, there is a need to evaluate the effectiveness of various techniques with the numerous types of concepts that exist (e.g., static, process, aesthetic, empirical concepts). For concept development to be effective, it should provide some release from ambiguity, enhance understanding, and provide direction for continuing development.

Other Applications for Concept Development Techniques

For the most part, we have focused this text on the contributions made to nursing knowledge and research through the use of concept development techniques. These contributions are quite significant in themselves. However, while expanding the knowledge base of the discipline through the resolution of significant problems is an admirable accomplishment, it does not constitute the only use of concept development techniques. We would not be providing a complete picture of the usefulness of concept development if we did not give some attention to these other applications, especially the use of these techniques to clarify ideas on an individual level and as a teaching strategy.

INDIVIDUAL CLARIFICATION OF IDEAS

In some respects, this application of concept development resembles the specific research uses of these methods discussed throughout this text. Although concept development may be an end point in itself when the purpose of inquiry is to clarify or expand a concept, it may also be an important preliminary step in an investigation. The use of concept development in this manner goes beyond the heuristic nature of some applications to assisting in the initial conceptualization of a study. In other cases, such methods have value simply for clarifying thoughts for future scholarly work.

Selecting and defining the appropriate concepts can be a difficult task in the early stages of a study. Yet, it is one of the most significant activities, ultimately affecting everything else in the investigation. For example, research on older adults' return to home after discharge from a hospital might be shaped much differently if the focus were on adaptation, coping, or integration (Westra & Rodgers, 1991). Similarly, Knafl and Deatrick (1987) found that conceptualizing family response to illness in regard to management, rather than the impact of the illness, directed their focus to very different aspects of the experience. These investigators successfully used concept analysis techniques to clarify and refine the concept of family management style (Deatrick & Knafl, 1990; Knafl & Deatrick, 1990). Concept development techniques can be very beneficial in identifying the appropriate focus to generate productive inquiry through clarifying or defining concepts or evaluating the fit of certain concepts with the situation of interest. These approaches may contribute to the development of a useful and coherent definition of key concepts in research, thereby helping the investigator avoid arbitrary or ad hoc definitions. Since methodological rigor and the usefulness of study findings may rest on the definitions used in a study, the contributions of concept development in the initial phases of an investigation cannot be underestimated.

Synthesizing vast amounts of literature, as accomplished through many of the concept development techniques, can be an important task in clarifying individual ideas as well. It is not uncommon for researchers, especially upon entering a new area of interest, to experience some confusion sorting through what may be multiple, diverse approaches to the subject matter. At such times it can be difficult to deal with these often conflicting ideas and either assimilate them into a coherent whole or develop a sound basis for choosing among competing ideas. Frequently, concept development techniques can provide a solid basis for presenting arguments regarding new ways to view a situation or innovative conceptualizations. Anyone who has worked with new investigators as they became mired in the confusion of the initial research stages, or who has had such an experience as they embarked on a new area of inquiry themselves, will recognize the value of concept development strategies for such purposes. We have recommended various concept development techniques on many occasions to students who were experiencing difficulty identifying a research focus, with overwhelmingly positive results.

Such activities have tremendous value in providing a strong basis for research and assisting in critical thought. Interestingly, concept development techniques, especially concept analysis, are becoming incorporated into graduate education in nursing with increasing frequency, perhaps for these very reasons. However, such activities may also account for the misconception that concept development constitutes merely an "academic exercise" (Diers, 1991). Consequently, we want to stress that the benefits and applications of such techniques extend well beyond academic or intellectual interests, as is evident in this text.

CONCEPT DEVELOPMENT IN TEACHING

The contributions of concept development techniques to the clarification of ideas is relevant even outside the context of actual research, particularly in their use as a teaching strategy. Indeed, Wilson's (1963) well-known work on concept analysis was developed for precisely this purpose. In 1988, Balog described his adaptation of the activities of concept analysis to assist health education students to explore and construct their own views of "health." Initially he provided the student group with a list of people of varying abilities and physical or medical conditions (e.g., athlete, person with myopia, paraplegic, person with bronchogenic carcinoma). The students were directed to explain if each hypothetical person on the list was *healthy* or *ill*. Ultimately, the class as a whole constructed lists of the "ingredients" for both the concepts of health and illness and worked to identify the essential criteria for each. This exercise not only assisted the students to construct their own views of health and illness but also, because of the group work involved, enhanced the students' awareness and appreciation of the wide scope of perspectives that individuals possess on this subject.

Other applications of concept development techniques in teaching are in the promotion of critical or analytical thinking. Students can be encouraged to confront key concepts in nursing by adapting some of the concept development strategies. On the undergraduate level, important concepts in nursing, such as the definition of nursing itself, professionalism, competence, collaboration, disease, human response, and diagnosis, can be explored using some of these techniques to help students come to grips with these ideas, obtain a depth of understanding of these concepts, and present a coherent presentation of their profession to others. As students progress to levels of increased clinical involvement, and in graduate nursing education, concepts relevant to patient care situations may be explored in a similar manner. The techniques of concept development may be an effective practical exercise to promote some of the analytical and critical skills appropriate to higher learning and essential to expert nursing practice.

A strength of many of the concept development techniques is the literature review involved in the process. These techniques provide, in most cases, some structure or system for conducting an extensive, in-depth literature review on the concepts of interest. Class projects or papers might provide an opportunity for students to use these techniques, thus presenting the student with a challenge to view the concept from multiple perspectives and to develop an awareness of the diversity of ideas. The process of comparing, contrasting, and eventually synthesizing ideas is an excellent exercise to develop analytical skills. Finally, if students present their own conclusions regarding the concept in some form, they have the opportunity to develop skill in preparing logical arguments and defending their positions in a public forum. As an added benefit, students may be learning an important skill for later involvement in research activities, thus potentially taking some of the mystery out of the research process as well.

Rodgers has presented concept analysis to nurses in clinical settings to develop their awareness and appreciation of this and other types of research and, especially, to instill an attitude that they *can* make an important contribution to the knowledge base of nursing. The processes involved in concept development are in no way simple or easy, as they require considerable powers of reasoning and analytical skill to be carried out well. Nevertheless, they have been perceived by practitioners as less threatening and, therefore, more manageable than a traditional quasi-experimental or experimental investigation. Unfortunately for many clinicians with entry-level education, these more traditional approaches to research constitute the extent of their knowledge about nursing inquiry.

Tadd and Chadwick (1989) also emphasized the contribution of various analytical techniques in the academic setting. Their discussion included various forms of philosophical analysis and was not focused on concept development specifically. However, their discussion added further emphasis to the value of such methods in teaching, particularly for clarifying ideas, increasing awareness of diverse perspectives and the complexity of language, and promoting the development of analytical skills.

One additional dimension addressed by Tadd and Chadwick (1989) included the use of such techniques by faculty involved in curriculum development. As these authors point out, concepts may be "incorporated into nursing curricula without adequate analysis or indeed without asking rather obvious questions about justifying their inclusion" (p. 157). In many instances, it is unreasonable to expect nurse educators to have a consensus on the definitions of important concepts; certainly there is a need for students to develop a tolerance for ambiguity and diversity. In other situations, agreement is both important and possible, for example, agreement on the notion of competence (or, in another common phrase, "safe professional practice"), which may be a hallmark in the evaluation of student performance and progress. Still, Tadd and Chadwick's call for concentrated attention regarding concepts as they are included in nursing curricula sends a significant caution to nurse educators, and demonstrates yet another application of concept development techniques.

Only a few journal articles were found in which concept development techniques were discussed in reference to nursing education. However, even these limited examples demonstrated the value of these methods in the academic setting. As Dungog (1988) points out, "exploratory rather than expository strategies" may be very effective in promoting learning (p. 14) and in producing graduates capable of success in a constantly changing environment (Tadd & Chadwick, 1989).

Future Directions for Concept Development in Nursing

In a 1979 research conference presentation, Downs argued that

> [nurse researchers] have already hurtled into too much clinical and applied research without sufficient attention to the theory on which it is based. . . . Short shrift is given to efforts aimed at producing descriptive material that could result in the construction of sound experiments later on. (Downs, 1980, p. 97)

Several facts could point to the rejection of this quote as bearing any relevance to nursing research now. First, it was presented well over a decade ago, and a decade is a vast amount of time in discussions of scientific activities and, especially, in view of the development of nursing knowledge that has occurred during this interim. Second, Downs was referring specifically to evaluation research (the focus of the conference), and the lack of "some kind of unifying theory that will place the huge volume of findings into some kind of theoretical juxtaposition" (p. 94). Finally, although Downs did refer directly to theory development, she did not mention the role of concept development in this process.

We would argue that Downs' (1980) admonition is not the least bit misplaced in the context of contemporary nursing investigations. As the hue and cry for more intervention-oriented, outcome-focused research continues to gain volume, there is considerable danger that nurse researchers will not have a sound descriptive base for their research, and that conceptual problems will undermine the apparent success brought about in the resolution of empirical or clinical problems (Laudan, 1977). Consequently, the balance between empirical advance and conceptual clarity may be lost, and progress becomes illusory, mired in the new dilemmas that are created along the way.

PROVIDING A DESCRIPTIVE BASIS

Concept development techniques can provide an important part of this descriptive base through the various outcomes that are achieved with these methods: accomplishments of a linguistic, communicative, categorical or classificatory, diagnostic, and heuristic nature. The linguistic function emphasizes word use to clarify vocabulary and alternate forms of expression. The communicative aspect may focus on consensus building to improve understanding and the sharing of ideas. Classification constitutes an important function of concepts that, when the concepts are clarified, enable phenomena to be sorted or categorized relative to shared attributes. This process may be used particularly in the development of taxonomic structures, for example, the development of nursing diagnoses (Lunney, 1990). Finally, the heuristic potential of concept development techniques provides direction for further research by generating not only plausible definitions but questions and, sometimes, hypotheses for further research (Rodgers, 1989a, 1989b).

These functions point to the strong basis for further research that can result from the development of concepts. Yet, it is important to avoid constructing an apparent hierarchical notion of research, where description has value only if it leads later to empirical testing. Description is a valuable end point in itself, because of its power in illustrating or increasing sensitivity to experience, and enhancing understanding.

Furthermore, concept development techniques are not limited to description alone. At times, they border on the prescriptive (if we can use that term safely in this context), suggesting not how nurses *should act* or what they *should do,* but how nurses *might think* about a given situation or topic. It is difficult to argue against the merits of improved or, at least, expanded thinking! Of course, thinking is meant here to refer to the entire domain of cognitive activities. Improvement may take the form of clearly better (more useful, appropriate, or effective) ways to think about something or a challenge to the status quo. Both of these are important components of progress.

ATTENTION TO CONCEPTUAL PROBLEMS

New directions for concept development thus include the increased recognition of conceptual problems, the use of appropriate techniques for their resolution, and the continuing expansion and evaluation of methods, along with the creation of additional methods as new and unique types of problems are identified. In recent years, there has been a great deal of attention to (and, for the most part, support for) the idea of a balance in the generation of nursing knowledge. Typically, these discussions have focused on qualitative and quantitative methods as the entities to be weighed (Knafl, Pettengill, Bevis, & Kirchhoff, 1988; Morse, 1991). While these debates have some merit, we suggest that balance be considered not only in regard to the methods used. Instead, balance is needed among the types of knowledge that are generated and the kinds of problems solved. For our purposes here, we are concerned especially with the attention given to both empirical and conceptual problems. Throughout this text, there are numerous examples of conceptual problems that have a significant impact on nursing knowledge and practice and that, as a result, cannot be ignored in the scientific enterprise of nursing.

This idea of balance is not unlike the anecdote of sawing off the legs of a chair that sits unevenly on the floor. Nurse scholars must be careful that in resolving some problems, the new problems that will be created as a part of the process are not left unattended. More realistically, every problem "solved" undoubtedly will result in new questions. The task, then, is for inquiry to be pursued in a variety of realms, focused on diverse problems, and with methods appropriate to answer the questions deemed important in nursing. At the same time, it is important not only to recognize the contributions of these varied approaches, but to integrate and build upon their unique contributions.

Indeed, as editors, we might be viewed as having created a few additional problems with this book. One of our primary aims was to call attention to a class of problems that previously may have been misunderstood, inadequately recognized, thought to be incapable of resolution, perhaps ignored altogether, or, in some circumstances, given "second class" status. Calling attention to problems, however, seems to be prerequisite to making progress in an area. More important, we have provided a cross-section of valuable tools for addressing the problems that may be identified as a result of this work. We hope this text will contribute to increased understanding of these tools, a foundation for reasoned decision making in the design of investigations, and, ultimately, rigorous and defensible inquiry to promote continued, productive investigations. Our intent in this concluding chapter, then, was not to bring closure, but to open doors to enhance concept development in nursing.

REFERENCES

Balog, J. E. (1988). The concept of health and techniques of conceptual analysis. *Health Education, 19*(4), 54–56.

Deatrick, J., & Knafl, K. (1990). Family management behaviors: Concept analysis and refinement. *Journal of Pediatric Nursing, 5,* 15–22.

Diers, D. (1991). On academic exercises. . . . *Image: Journal of Nursing Scholarship, 23,* 70.

Downs, F. S. (1980). Relationship of findings of clinical research and development of criteria: A researcher's perspective. *Nursing Research, 29,* 94–97.

Dungog, E. F. (1988). Concept teaching in nursing. *ANPhi Papers, 23*(1), 12–14.

Knafl, K. A., & Deatrick, J. A. (1987). Conceptualizing family response to a child's chronic illness or disability. *Family Relations, 36,* 300–304.

Knafl, K. A., & Deatrick, J. A. (1990). Family management style: Concept analysis and development. *Journal of Pediatric Nursing, 5,* 4–14.

Knafl, K., Pettengill, M., Bevis, M., & Kirchhoff, K. (1988). Blending qualitative and quantitative approaches to instrument development and data collection. *Journal of Professional Nursing, 4,* 30–37.

Laudan, L. (1977). *Progress and its problems.* Berkeley: University of California Press.

Lunney, M. (1990). Accuracy of nursing diagnoses: Concept development. *Nursing Diagnosis, 1*(1), 12–17.

Morse, J. M. (1991). *Qualitative nursing research: A contemporary dialogue* (rev. ed.). Newbury Park, Calif: Sage.

Rodgers, B. L. (1989a). Concepts, analysis, and the development of nursing knowledge: The evolutionary cycle. *Journal of Advanced Nursing, 14,* 330–335.

Rodgers, B. L. (1989b). Exploring health policy as a concept. *Western Journal of Nursing Research, 11,* 694–702.

Tadd, W., & Chadwick, R. (1989). Philosophical analysis and its value to the nurse teacher. *Nurse Education Today, 9,* 155–160.

Westra, B. L., & Rodgers, B. L. (1991). The concept of integration: A foundation for evaluating outcomes of nursing care. *Journal of Professional Nursing, 7,* 277–282.

Wilson, J. (1963). *Thinking with concepts.* London: Cambridge University Press.

Bibliography

This bibliography represents a broad cross-section of literature with relevance to concept development in nursing. A variety of viewpoints can be found in this literature, which is drawn primarily from philosophy, psychology, nursing, and other health sciences. The works included here were selected primarily for their contribution to understanding the notion of *concepts* in general, and diverse approaches to concept development, along with discussions of specific concepts of interest in nursing.

Arakelian, M. (1980). An assessment and nursing application of the concept of locus of control. *Advances in Nursing Science, 3*(1), 25–42.

Armstrong, S. L., Gleitman, L. R., & Gleitman, H. (1983). What some concepts might not be. *Cognition, 13,* 263–308.

Artinian, B. (1982). Conceptual mapping: Development of the strategy. *Western Journal of Nursing Research, 4,* 379–393.

Avant, K. (1979). Nursing diagnosis: Maternal attachment. *Advances in Nursing Science, 2*(1), 45–55.

Avant, K. C. (1991). Paths to concept development in nursing diagnosis. *Nursing Diagnosis, 2*(3), 105–110.

Balog, J. E. (1982). The concept of health and disease: A relativistic perspective. *Health Values: Achieving High Level Wellness, 6*(5), 7–13.

Balog, J. E. (1988). The concept of health and techniques of conceptual analysis. *Health Education, 19*(4), 54–56.

Barsalou, L. W., & Medin, D. L. (1986). Concepts: Static definitions or context-dependent representations? *Cahiers de Psychologie Cognitive, 6,* 187–202.

Battenfield, B. L. (1984). Suffering: A conceptual description and content analysis of an operational schema. *Image: Journal of Nursing Scholarship, 16,* 36–41.

Beck, C. T. (1982). The conceptualization of power. *Advances in Nursing Science, 4*(2), 1–17.

Becker, C. H. (1983). A conceptualization of concept. *Nursing Papers, 15*(2), 51–58.

Beeber, L. S., & Schmitt, M. H. (1986). Cohesiveness in groups: A concept in search of a definition. *Advances in Nursing Science, 8*(2), 1–11.

Berthold, J. S. (1964). Theoretical and empirical clarification of concepts. *Nursing Science, 2,* 406–422.

Beyea, S. C. (1990). Concept analysis of feeling: A human response pattern. *Nursing Diagnosis, 1*(3), 97–101.

Bloch, D. (1974). Some crucial terms in nursing: What do they really mean? *Nursing Outlook, 22,* 689–694.

Bolton, N. (1977). *Concept formation.* New York: Pergamon Press.

Boyd, C. (1985). Toward an understanding of mother-daughter identification using concept analysis. *Advances in Nursing Science, 7*(3), 78–86.

Brooks, J. A., & Kleine-Kracht, A. E. (1983). Evolution of a definition of nursing. *Advances in Nursing Science, 5*(4), 51–68.

Brownell, M. J. (1984). The concept of crisis: Its utility for nursing. *Advances in Nursing Science, 6*(3), 10–21.

Brubaker, B. H. (1983). Health promotion: A linguistic analysis. *Advances in Nursing Science, 5*(3), 1–14.

Burkhardt, M. A. (1989). Spirituality: An analysis of the concept. *Holistic Nursing Practice, 3*(3), 69–77.

Campbell, L. (1987). Hopelessness: A concept analysis. *Journal of Psychosocial Nursing and Mental Health Services, 25*(2), 18–22.

Capers, C. F. (1986). Some basic facts about models, nursing conceptualizations, and nursing theories. *Journal of Continuing Education in Nursing, 16*(5), 149–154.

Carlson-Sabelli, L. (1989). Role reversal: A concept analysis and reinterpretation of the research literature. *Journal of Group Psychotherapy, Psychodrama & Sociometry, 41*(4), 139–152.

Carnap, R. (1956). *Meaning and necessity.* Chicago: University of Chicago Press.

Carnes, B. A. (1984). Concept analysis: Dependence. *Critical Care Quarterly, 6*(4), 29–39.

Chinn, P. L., & Jacobs, M. (1987). *Theory and nursing: A systematic approach* (2nd ed.). St. Louis: Mosby.

Chinn, P. L., & Kramer, M. (1991). *Theory and nursing: A systematic approach* (3rd ed.). St. Louis: Mosby.

Cowles, K. V. (1984). Life, death, and personhood. *Nursing Outlook, 32,* 169–172.

Cowles, K. V., & Rodgers, B. L. (1991). The concept of grief: A foundation for nursing practice and research. *Research in Nursing and Health, 14,* 119–127.

Crawford, G. (1982). The concept of patterns in nursing: Conceptual development and measurement. *Advances in Nursing Science, 5*(4), 1–6.

de Jong-Gierveld, J. (1989). Personal relationships, social support, and loneliness. *Journal of Social and Personal Relationships, 6,* 197–221.

Dolfman, M. L. (1973). The concept of health: An historic and analytic examination. *Journal of School Health, 43,* 491–497.

Dubin, R. (1969). *Theory building.* New York: Free Press.

Duffy, M. E. (1987). The concept of adaptation: Examining alternatives for the study of nursing phenomena. *Scholarly Inquiry for Nursing Practice, 1,* 179–192.

Duldt, B. W., & Giffin, K. (1985). *Theoretical perspectives for nursing.* Boston: Little, Brown.

Edel, A. (1979). *Analyzing concepts in social science.* New Brunswick, NJ: Transaction Books.

Engelmann, S. (1969). *Conceptual learning.* Belmont, Calif: Dimensions.

Epstein, S. (1973). The self-concept revisited or a theory of a theory. *American Psychologist, 28,* 404–416.

Evans, S. K. (1979). Descriptive criteria for the concept of depleted health potential. *Advances in Nursing Science, 1*(3), 67–74.

Fawcett, J. (1989). *Analysis and evaluation of conceptual models of nursing* (2nd ed.). Norwalk, Conn: Appleton & Lange.

Fehr, B. (1988). Prototype analysis of the concepts of love and commitment. *Journal of Personality and Social Psychology, 55,* 557–579.

Field, E. R. (1980). Authority: A select power. *Advances in Nursing Science, 3*(1), 69–83.

Flew, A. (Ed.) (1960). *Essays in Conceptual Analysis.* London: Macmillan.

Forsyth, G. L. (1980). Analysis of the concept of empathy: Illustration of one approach. *Advances in Nursing Science, 2*(2), 33–42.

Friedemann, M. L. (1989). The concept of family nursing. *Journal of Advanced Nursing, 14,* 211–216.

Geach, P., & Black, M. (Eds.) (1970). *Translations from the philosophical writings of Gottlob Frege.* Oxford: Basil Blackwell.

Gibbs, J. P. (1972). *Sociological theory construction.* Hinsdale, Ill: Dryden.

Gibson, C. H. (1991). A concept analysis of empowerment. *Journal of Advanced Nursing, 16,* 354–361.

Gillett, G. R. (1987). Concepts, structures, and meanings. *Inquiry, 30,* 101–112.

Goosen, G. M. (1989). Concept analysis: An approach to teaching physiologic variables. *Journal of Professional Nursing, 5*(1), 31–38.

Gordon, M. (1990). Toward theory-based diagnostic categories. *Nursing Diagnosis, 1*(1), 5–11.

Green, J. A. (1979). Science, nursing, and nursing science: A conceptual analysis. *Advances in Nursing Science, 2*(1), 57-64.

Griffin, A. P. (1983). A philosophical analysis of caring in nursing. *Journal of Advanced Nursing, 8,* 289–295.

Haight, B. K., & Warren, J. (1991). Apathy: Development of a nursing diagnosis. *Applied Nursing Research, 4,* 186–187.

Hardy, M. E. (1973). *Theoretical foundations for nursing.* New York: MSS Information.

Hardy, M. E. (1974). Theories: Components, development, evaluation. *Nursing Research, 23,* 100–107.

Hawks, J. H. (1991). Power: A concept analysis. *Journal of Advanced Nursing, 16,* 754–762.

Hempel, C. G. (1952). *Fundamentals of concept formation in empirical science.* Chicago: University of Chicago Press.

Henry, C. (1987). Persons and humans. *Journal of Advanced Nursing, 12,* 383–388.

Henry, C., & Tuxill, A. C. (1987). Concept of the person: Introduction to the health professionals. *Journal of Advanced Nursing, 12,* 245–249.

Hinds, P. S. (1984). Inducing a definition of hope through the use of grounded theory methodology. *Journal of Advanced Nursing, 9,* 357–362.

Jones, J. A. (1983). Where angels fear to tread—nursing and the concept of creativity. *Journal of Advanced Nursing, 8,* 405–411.

Jones, P. S. (1985). Developing concepts and conceptual frameworks in nursing. *ANPhi Papers, 20*(1-2), 8–14.

Kahn, D. L., & Steeves, R. H. (1986). The experience of suffering: Conceptual clarification and theoretical definition. *Journal of Advanced Nursing, 11,* 623–631.

Kane, C. F. (1988). Family social support: Toward a conceptual model. *Advances in Nursing Science, 10*(2), 18–25.

Kaplan, A. (1964). *The conduct of inquiry* (2nd ed.). St. Louis: Mosby.

Keck, J. F. (1986). Terminology of theory development. In A. Marriner (Ed.), *Nursing theorists and their work* (pp. 15–23). St. Louis: Mosby.

Keller, M. J. (1981). Toward a definition of health. *Advances in Nursing Science, 4,* 43–64.

Kemp, V. H. (1985). Concept analysis as a strategy for promoting critical thinking. *Journal of Nursing Education, 24,* 382–384.

Kerr, N. J. (1985). Behavioral manifestations of misguided entitlement. *Perspectives in Psychiatric Care, 23*(1), 5–15.

Kim, H. S. (1983). *The nature of theoretical thinking in nursing.* Norwalk, Conn: Appleton-Century-Crofts.

King, I. M. (1975). A process for developing concepts for nursing through research. In P. Verhonick (Ed.), *Nursing Research I* (pp. 25–43). Boston: Little, Brown.

King, I. M. (1988). Concepts: Essential elements of theories. *Nursing Science Quarterly, 1*(1), 22–25.

Kleinpell, R. M. (1991). Concept analysis of quality of life. *Dimensions of Critical Care Nursing, 10,* 223–229.

Knafl, K. A., & Deatrick, J. A. (1986). How families manage chronic conditions: An analysis of the concept of normalization. *Research in Nursing and Health, 9,* 215–222.

Knafl K. A., & Deatrick, J. A. (1990). Family management style: Concept analysis and development. *Journal of Pediatric Nursing, 5*(1), 4–14.

Kolcaba, K. Y., & Kolcaba, R. J. (1991). An analysis of the concept of comfort. *Journal of Advanced Nursing, 16,* 1301–1310.

Kripke, S. A. (1980). *Naming and necessity.* Oxford: Basil Blackwell.

Laudan, L. (1977). *Progress and its problems.* Berkeley: University of California Press.

Lee, H. J. (1983). Analysis of a concept: Hardiness. *Oncology Nursing Forum, 10*(4), 32–35.

Lemone, P. (1991). Analysis of a human phenomenon: Self-concept. *Nursing Diagnosis, 2*(3), 126–130.

Lindgren, C. L., Burke, M. L., Hainsworth, M. A., & Eakes, G. G. (1992). Chronic sorrow: A lifespan concept. *Scholarly Inquiry for Nursing Practice, 6*(1), 27–40.

Lindsey, E., & Hills, M. (1992). An analysis of the concept of hardiness. *Canadian Journal of Nursing Research, 24*(1), 39–50.

Lunney, M. (1990). Accuracy of nursing diagnoses: Concept development. *Nursing Diagnosis, 1*(1), 12–17.

Madden, B. P. (1990). The hybrid model for concept development: Its value for the study of therapeutic alliance. *Advances in Nursing Science, 12*(3), 75–87.

Matteson, P., & Hawkins, J. W. (1990). Concept analysis of decision-making. *Nursing Forum, 25*(2), 4–10.

McCloskey, M. E., & Glucksberg, S. (1978). Natural categories: Well defined or fuzzy sets? *Memory & Cognition, 6,* 462–472.

Medin, D. L. (1989). Concepts and conceptual structure. *American Psychologist, 44,* 1469–1481.

Medin, D. L., & Schaffer, M. M. (1978). Context theory of classification learning. *Psychological Review, 85,* 207–238.

Medin, D. L., & Smith, E. E. (1984). Concepts and concept formation. *Annual Review of Psychology, 35,* 113–138.

Meize-Grochowski, R. (1984). An analysis of the concept of trust. *Journal of Advanced Nursing, 9,* 563–572.

Meleis, A. I. (1985). *Theoretical nursing.* Philadelphia: Lippincott.

Moch, S. D. (1989). Health within illness: Conceptual evolution and practice possibilities. *Advances in Nursing Science, 11*(4), 23–31.

Morse, J. M., Bottorff, J., Neander, W., & Solberg, S. (1991). Comparative analysis of conceptualizations and theories of caring. *Image: Journal of Nursing Scholarship, 23,* 119–126.

Morse, J. M., Solberg, S. M., Neander, W. L., Bottorff, J. L., & Johnson, J. L. (1990). Concepts of caring and caring as a concept. *Advances in Nursing Science, 13*(1), 1–14.

Nemcek, M. A. (1987). Self nurturing: A concept analysis. *AAOHN Journal, 35,* 349–352.

Norris, C. M. (1982). *Concept clarification in nursing.* Rockville, Md: Aspen.

Nursing Development Conference Group. (1979). *Concept formalization in nursing* (2nd ed.). Boston: Little, Brown.

Oleson, M. (1990). Subjectively perceived quality of life. *Image: Journal of Nursing Scholarship, 22,* 187–190.

Osherson, D. N., & Smith, E. E. (1981). On the adequacy of prototype theory as a theory of concepts. *Cognition, 9,* 35–58.

Panzarine, S. (1985). Coping: Conceptual and methodological issues. *Advances in Nursing Science, 7,* 49–58.

Parse, R. R. (1987). *Nursing science: Major paradigms, theories, and critiques.* Philadelphia: W.B. Saunders.

Payne, L. (1983). Health: A basic concept in nursing theory. *Journal of Advanced Nursing, 8,* 393–395.

Potempa, K., Lopez, M., Reid, C., & Lawson, L. (1986). Chronic fatigue. *Image: Journal of Nursing Scholarship, 18*(4), 165–169.

Price, H. H. (1953). *Thinking and experience.* London: Hutchinson House.

Putnam, H. (1957). Psychological concepts, explication, and ordinary language. *Journal of Philosophy, 54,* 94–100.

Putnam, H. (1975). *Mind, language, and reality: Philosophical papers* (Vol. 2). Cambridge: Cambridge University Press.

Quine, W. V. D. (1960). *Word and object.* Cambridge, Mass: MIT Press.

Rawnsley, M. M. (1980). The concept of privacy. *Advances in Nursing Science, 2,* 25–31.

Rawnsley, M. M. (1980). Toward a conceptual base for affective nursing. *Nursing Outlook, 28,* 244–247.

Rawnsley, M. M. (1985). Nursing: The compassionate science. *Cancer Nursing* (Supplement 1), *8,* 71–74.

Reed, P. G., & Leonard, V. E. (1989). An analysis of the concept of self-neglect. *Advances in Nursing Science, 12*(1), 39–53.

Rew, L. (1986). Intuition: Concept analysis of a group phenomenon. *Advances in Nursing Science, 8*(2), 21–28.

Rew, L., & Barrow, E. M. (1987). Intuition: A neglected hallmark of nursing knowledge. *Advances in Nursing Science, 10*(1), 49–62.

Reynolds, P. D. (1971). *A primer in theory construction.* New York: Bobbs-Merrill.

Rodgers, B. L. (1989). Concepts, analysis, and the development of nursing knowledge: The evolutionary cycle. *Journal of Advanced Nursing, 14,* 330–335.

Rodgers, B. L. (1989). Exploring health policy as a concept. *Western Journal of Nursing Research, 11,* 694–702.

Rodgers, B. L. (1989). The use and application of concepts in nursing: The case of health policy. (Doctoral dissertation, University of Virginia, 1987). *Dissertation Abstracts International, 49*–11B, 4756.

Rodgers, B. L. (1991). Using concept analysis to enhance clinical practice and research. *Dimensions of Critical Care Nursing, 10*(1), 28–34.

Rodgers, B. L., & Cowles, K. V. (1991). The concept of grief: An analysis of classical and contemporary thought. *Death Studies, 15,* 443–458.

Rosch, E., & Mervis, C. B. (1975). Family resemblances: Studies in the internal structure of categories. *Cognitive Psychology, 7,* 573–605.

Rosenbaum, J. N. (1989). Self-caring: Concept development for nursing. *Recent Advances in Nursing, 24,* 18–31.

Ryle, G. (1949). *The concept of mind.* Chicago: University of Chicago Press.

Ryle, G. (1971). *Collected papers* (Vols. 1–2). London: Hutchinson House.

Sarkis, J. M., & Skoner, M. M. (1987). An analysis of the concept of holism in nursing literature. *Holistic Nursing Practice, 2*(1), 61–69.

Sartori, G. (1984). *Social science concepts: A systematic analysis.* Beverly Hills: Sage.

Schwartz-Barcott, D., & Kim, H. S. (1986). A hybrid model for concept development. In P. L. Chinn (Ed.). *Nursing Research Methodology: Issues and Implementation* (pp. 91–101). Rockville, Md: Aspen.

Simmons, S. J. (1989). Health: A concept analysis. *International Journal of Nursing Studies, 26,* 155–161.

Smith, J. A. (1981). The idea of health: A philosophical inquiry. *Advances in Nursing Science, 3*(3), 43–50.

Sokal, R. R. (1974). Classification: Purposes, principles, progress, prospects. *Science, 185,* 1115–1123.

Sokolowski, R. L. (1987). Exorcising concepts. *The Review of Metaphysics, 40,* 451–463.

Soltis, J. (1978). *An introduction to the analysis of educational concepts.* Reading, Pa: Addison-Wesley.

Stephenson, C. (1991). The concept of hope revisited for nursing. *Journal of Advanced Nursing, 16,* 1456–1461.

Stevens, B. (1984). *Nursing theory: Analysis, application and evaluation* (2nd ed.). Boston: Little, Brown.

Sullivan, T. D. (1982). Concepts. *New Scholasticism, 56,* 146–168.

Summers, I., Coffelt, T., & Horton, R. E. (1988). Work-group cohesion. *Psychological Reports,* *63,* 627–636.

Tadd, W., & Chadwick, R. (1989). Philosophical analysis and its value to the nurse teacher. *Nurse Education Today, 9,* 155–160.

Teasdale, K. (1989). The concept of reassurance in nursing. *Journal of Advanced Nursing,* *14,* 444–450.

Teel, C. S. (1991). Chronic sorrow: Analysis of the concept. *Journal of Advanced Nursing,* *16,* 1311–1319.

Timmerman, C. M. (1991). A concept analysis of intimacy. *Issues in Mental Health Nursing,* *12*(1), 19–30.

Toulmin, S. (1972). *Human understanding.* Princeton, NJ: Princeton University Press.

Trandel-Korenchuck, D. M. (1986). Concept development in nursing research. *Nursing Administration Quarterly, 11*(1), 1–9.

Vincent, P. (1975). Some crucial terms in nursing—A second opinion. *Nursing Outlook,* *23*(1), 46–48.

Watson, J. (1985). *Nursing: Human science and human care.* Norwalk, Conn: Appleton-Century-Crofts.

Watson, S. J. (1991). An analysis of the concept of experience. *Journal of Advanced Nursing,* *16,* 1117–1121.

Weitz, M. (1977). *The opening mind.* Chicago: University of Chicago Press.

Westra, B. L., & Rodgers, B. L. (1991). The concept of intergration: A foundation for evaluating outcomes of nursing care. *Journal of Professional Nursing, 7,* 277–282.

Whitley, G. G. (1992). Concept analysis of anxiety. *Nursing Diagnosis, 3,* 107–116.

Whitley, G. G. (1992). Concept analysis of fear. *Nursing Diagnosis, 3,* 155–161.

Wilson, J. (1963). *Thinking with concepts.* London: Cambridge University Press.

Wilson, J. (1985). The inevitability of certain concepts (including education): A reply to Robin Barrow. *Educational Theory, 35,* 203–204.

Wittgenstein, L. (1968). *Philosophical investigations* (3rd ed.) (G. E. M. Anscombe, Trans.). New York: Macmillan. (Original work published 1953)

Wittgenstein, L. (1981). *Tractatus Logico-philosophicus* (D. F. Pears & B. F. McGuiness, Trans.). Great Britain: Whitstable Litho. (Original work published 1921)

Yoder, L. (1990). Mentoring: A concept analysis. *Nursing Administration Quarterly, 15*(1), 9–19.

Yolton, J. W. (1960). Concept analysis. *Kantstudien, 52,* 467–484.

Younger, J. B. (1991). A theory of mastery. *Advances in Nursing Science, 14*(1), 76–89.

Index

Note: Page numbers in *italics* refer to figures; page numbers followed by a (t) refer to tables.

A

A priori concepts, 15
Abstraction, 12, 14
Acceptance, concept of, 178
   critical attributes of, 186
   definition of, 182
Adaptation, concept of, 129(t)
Advocacy, concept of, 127, 128(t)
AIDSLINE, 200(t)
Alienation, concept of, 129(t)
Alliance, therapeutic, concept of, 128(t)
Anaclitic depression, 137
Analysis, unit of, 115-116
Analytical thinking, concept development
   in, 238
Anger, concept of, 116
Anguish, concept of, 124, 129(t)
Annotation, in literature search, 202-206,
   203(t)-204(t), 205(t)
Anomie, concept of, 129(t)
Anxiety, concept of, 129
  nursing diagnosis of, 228-229
  separation, concept of, 129(t)
  underlying, in Wilson method, 58, 70
Apathy reaction, 138
Aristotle, 12
Assigning, act of, in delegation, 62
Attachment, concept of, 128(t)
Attributes, essential, 19-20
Authority, in concept of delegation, 62
Autonomy, concept of, 129(t)
Avant, K. C., 43-44, 225-226

B

Bereavement, 94-95, 98, 102. See also *Grief.*
BIOETHICSLINE, 200(t)

BIOSIS, 200(t)
Body image, concept of, 129(t)
Bonding, concept of, 127, 128(t)
   contrary case for, 117-118, 120
   model case for, 116-117, 120
   related case for, 122-123
   touch in, 120
   voice quality in, 120
Boredom, concept of, 129(t)
Brief Psychiatric Rating Scale, in withdrawal
   measurement, 141

C

Cancer, terminal, anguish of, 124
CANCERLINE, 199, 200(t)
Care providers, grief consequences for, 101
Caring, concept of, 120-121, 127, 128(t)
Case(s), borderline, in concept clarification,
   47
   in hybrid model, 116, 121-122
   in Wilson method, 56-57, 67-68
  contrary, 116
   in concept clarification, 47
   in hybrid model, 116, 117-118, 120-
    121
   in Wilson method, 55-56, 64-65
  exemplary, 39, 43
  in hybrid model, 115-118, 145-146
  invented, in Wilson method, 57, 68-69
  model, 116
   in concept clarification, 47
   in evolutionary analysis, 86-87
   in hybrid model, 116, 119-120
   in Wilson method, 54-55, 63-64
  related, 84, 116
   in concept clarification, 47

249